# It's *NOT* Just Baby Fat!

## 10 Steps to Help Your Child to a Healthy Weight

Edward Abramson, Ph.D.

**Bodega Books**
**Lafayette, California**

**Ordering Information**

**Quantity Sales.** Special discounts are available on quantity sales. For information contact Bodega Books at the address above.

**Individual Sales.** Additional copies of *It's NOT Just Baby Fat!* can be ordered from the publisher at the above address or online at: www.itsnotjustbabyfat.com

Library of Congress Control Number: 2010917210

ISBN-13: 978-0-615-42075-2
ISBN-10: 0-615-42075-3

Printed in the United States of America

This book presents information based on research and the clinical experience of the author. It is not intended to be a substitute for personal consultation with a medical or psychological professional. The author and publisher disclaim liability for any adverse effects resulting directly or indirectly from information contained in this book.

# Preface

Several people offered support and help throughout the process of writing this book. Although I initially claimed that I didn't have the time to write another book, Roberta Guise convinced me otherwise. Now that it's finished I have to admit that she was right and I was wrong. Dr. Ann Steiner encouraged my speaking career while Nancy Bennett, R.D.A. and Dr. Ben Bernstein graciously offered advice on publishing. Denise Zetterbaum read the first draft of every chapter and offered suggestions that clarified and improved the wording, while Kathleen Marusak did an excellent job copy editing the manuscript.

As you read the book, it will be obvious that I couldn't have written it without the examples that so many of my clients, students, and workshop participants have provided. While I've changed the identifying details of their stories, the insights I've gained from working with them permeate the book. I'm grateful to them for sharing part of their lives with me.

Finally, I need to acknowledge Jeremy, Annie, Sam, and Bessie. You guys are great!

# Table of Contents

# Part I: It's NOT Just Baby Fat

Allow me to introduce myself. I was a fat kid. I wore "husky" clothes and was called "chubby." I had a sweet tooth: cookies with lunch, more cookies with milk when I came home from school, chocolate sneaked from my mother's stash late in the afternoon and ice cream for dessert every night. Although I rode my bicycle, I generally preferred sitting to moving and avoided anything athletic. In sixth grade, when my dad tried to sign me up for Little League, I complained until he relented. In high school I volunteered to be the attendance monitor in gym class so that I could avoid actually doing anything strenuous.

When I got to college I slimmed down a little but still avoided anything requiring significant physical exertion. By the time I was in my early 30's, I was again overweight and on my way to becoming obese. Since my mother and my brother were both obese, I figured it was in my genes and there was little I could do about it. I was wrong, there was plenty I could do about it. The premature deaths of my mother and brother from obesity-related causes greatly intensified my interest in losing weight.

Currently I weigh 15 pounds less than I did as a young adult and I'm in far better shape. Since Americans gain an average of over one pound a year throughout adulthood, if I hadn't done anything my BMI would have been over 30 by now, placing me in the obese category. Although I've been successful in losing weight, it would have been far easier to avoid the weight gain as a child. I could have learned the healthy habits that would have allowed me to maintain a normal weight instead of going through the difficult process of unlearning the unhealthy habits.

In graduate school my personal interest and a fortuitous meeting with a psychology professor, who had an obesity research grant, led to my dissertation research on emotions and eating. I was hooked — I've been involved in treating, conducting research, lecturing, and writing about obesity and eating disorders ever since.

For several years I was the director of a hospital-based weight loss program. Many of the participants talked about difficulties they were having with their overweight kids:

- "Should I worry about my son's weight or is it just baby fat that he'll outgrow?"
- "When my daughter comes home from school, she just stays in her room and watches TV. Is that normal?"
- "My son just likes junk food. How do I get him to eat vegetables?"
- "My nine-year-old daughter needs to lose weight. Can I bring her in to see you?"

The hospital program was not set up to provide direct services to children but I was able to provide some guidance for their parents. As it turns out, research has demonstrated that overweight children don't benefit from direct treatment, but parents can be very effective in helping their kids lose weight.

Even if your child is the only one in the family that is overweight, helping him lose the weight requires the whole family's involvement. You can't just single out the overweight child for special treatment; everyone should be involved. Putting a child on a diet and telling him to exercise while the rest of the family is eating ice cream and watching TV won't work, but if the whole family participates everyone will benefit. The 10 Steps will help your child to achieve a healthy weight. If you've been dealing with your own weight issues, you'll find that most of the steps, with a little modification, will help with your struggle. This book will present the 10 Steps and show you how to follow them.

## If You've Been Struggling With Your Weight

If you're overweight or have been dieting you know how difficult weight loss can be. While you want to spare your child the difficulties you've had, you may be skeptical about the likelihood of success. You know that, despite the advertising claims, dieting rarely works. Yet, even with the gloomy statistics for adults, the good news is that weight loss is easier for children and doesn't require dieting.

Kids have several advantages over adults. The most obvious is that they're still growing and this process requires large amounts of energy. If you can help your child maintain his current weight, he will be less overweight as his height increases. Following the 10 Steps will help prevent your child from increasing energy intake (eating too much), while the natural growth will consume much of the excess energy he has stored (fat). The result will be a taller and leaner kid.

Another advantage that kids have over adults is that they enjoy playing. While you may find it difficult to "get motivated" to exercise, most younger kids don't need extra motivation to play. They'll play whenever they have the chance. If they're not watching TV or using a computer, most of their play will involve moving and burning calories. Follow Step 9 and your child will spend less time with TV and computers and more time in active play.

Many adults spend most of their day sitting — working at a desk, driving their car, or relaxing in front of the TV.

Kids, even when they're in school, spend less time sitting. Younger kids have recess, older kids change classes, so even if your child isn't in a gym class, he's probably moving more during the day. Step 8 will offer additional ideas to help your child keep moving.

Although the purpose of the 10 Steps is to help your child get to a healthy weight, you may find that as you implement the action plans for each step that you will start to lose. There aren't any rigid diets and most of the steps don't involve "will power," but rather changes in the household environment. You'll find that, by implementing these changes you will improve your eating and exercise habits. Even if you don't experience significant weight loss, you will be modeling the behaviors that will help your kids develop healthy habits. Although they might not admit it, kids, even rebellious teens, look up to their parents. When your children see you starting to change your habits, they'll be more motivated to follow through with the 10 Steps.

While reading this book should be informative, and hopefully interesting, the act of reading by itself will not produce any weight loss. To move from information to action I've included an action plan for each step. No child ever lost weight solely because his parents had good intentions. It's necessary to actually implement the action plans. Although you'll need to be persistent, you'll find they're not that difficult.

Before we get started, let me say something about gender. Most of the time I'll be writing about both boys and girls. Rather than use "he or she" every time, I've picked one or the other gender, but it applies equally to both. Where there are sex differences, the effects of early puberty, for example, I've made a point of specifying which gender I'm discussing.

# Chapter 1 –Baby Fat is the Beginning of Adult Fat

Julie S. was a chubby baby and toddler. When Julie started school, Mrs. S., who was on a diet, worried that Julie wouldn't outgrow her "baby fat." She started sharing her diet foods with her daughter. It didn't help; Julie continued to gain weight.

When Julie was in third grade, Mrs. S. felt that she had to get serious about Julie's weight so she put her on a diet, forbade junk foods, and set strict weight reduction goals for her. This didn't work either. Several times, Mrs. S. would catch Julie eating cookies, candy or other forbidden foods. "How many times do I have to tell you if you keep on eating cookies, you'll never lose weight?" Mrs. S. would yell. In a softer voice she would go on to say, "I'm so disappointed in you. You don't have any willpower. Don't you want to lose weight?" Sometimes, out of desperation, Mrs. S. threatened to punish Julie if she caught her eating junk foods again, but this didn't work either.

Julie has gone from being a chubby baby to being an overweight teen and then an obese adult. She is now 22 years old, five and a half feet tall, and weighs 195 pounds. What could Mrs. S. have done to prevent her chubby child from becoming obese? If you are concerned about your child's weight, what should you do?

Helping a child control his or her weight can be frustrating. Research shows that putting a child on a diet rarely works. More often it backfires. One study found that girls who frequently diet are 12 times as likely to be binge eaters! Like Julie, many kids on a diet actually gain more weight than equally heavy kids who don't diet. You may feel that you have to do something so that your son or daughter doesn't suffer as a fat child and become an obese adult. But what should you do?

Some parents aren't as focused on diets as Mrs. S. was yet they still encourage their children to lose weight. Consider Dan R.'s childhood. I met Dan when, at age 42, he called me for a psychological evaluation prior to bariatric surgery. Almost all surgeons require an evaluation before performing weight loss surgery to insure that the patient isn't depressed, suffering from an eating disorder or mental illness.

Dan was a chubby kid, but he wasn't bothered by his weight. With a sad expression on his face, he told me about an incident that occurred in his childhood:

> When I was nine I went boating with my father and stepmother. It was hot so I took my shirt off. My stepmother, who was always concerned about my weight, took my picture. The next week, when the photos were developed, she showed me the picture, pointed out how fat I was and gave me a lecture about losing weight. I was devastated.

As an adult Dan was 5 feet, 8 inches tall and weighed 265 pounds. He had a lot going for him. A "take-charge guy," he was a successful entrepreneur, having started two high tech firms in Silicon Valley. He was happily married and was the father of two young children. Despite his success in the other areas of his life, Dan just couldn't seem to lose weight, and it wasn't for lack of trying. He had been to Weight Watchers several times, tried Atkins, South Beach and countless other diets, been prescribed Meridia, a weight loss drug, and joined a gym, but to no avail. With some embarrassment he admitted that in his early 20's he'd had a bout of bulimia, but that just made him more miserable. He was desperate to lose so he was going in for surgery.

Parents try to do what's best for their kids: they want them to develop healthy habits so they use what they know, frequently what they've heard from their parents, to direct the child's behavior.

Parents make rules and offer advice. Have you ever told your kids:

- "Eat your vegetables if you want to grow up to be big and strong."
- "Turn off the TV and go out and get some exercise."
- "You can't have dessert unless you finish your vegetables."
- "If you don't lose some weight, no boy (girl) is going to be interested in you."

Or, if your advice and encouragement doesn't work, perhaps you've decided that more serious action is needed. Have you:

- Prohibited "junk food" or certain snacks;
- Put your child on a diet;
- Signed your child up for soccer, Little League or other sport activity hoping that it would help your child lose weight; or
- Enrolled your child in a weight loss program?

When you've tried these strategies, what happened? Often it seems that the parent and the child are engaged in a never-ending battle over what to eat or not eat, and unfortunately the child temporarily "wins" this battle. The child gains weight while the parents are frustrated and feel helpless. It doesn't have to be like this.

I will show you how Moms and Dads can avoid fights over food and weight and help their kids develop healthy eating habits, become active, and feel good about their bodies. You'll be able to help your child maintain a healthy weight without all the conflict.

# Chapter 2 - Should You Be Concerned About Your Child's Weight?

You're probably aware that the number of overweight kids has increased dramatically — it's tripled since the 1960's. Childhood obesity is not just an American phenomenon, it's increasing throughout much of the world. Recently I was having lunch in an English tearoom. While I was eating my cottage pie (meat with mashed potatoes) and vegetables, the overweight child at the table next to me was ordering pancakes with chocolate syrup. In some parts of Africa there is more juvenile obesity than starvation.

Kids don't all develop at the same pace so it's hard to know if you should be concerned about their weight. You don't know if your child will go from being a chubby preschooler to a lanky third grader or if the baby fat is the first step leading to adult obesity. If you're not sure, you've got plenty of company. Research suggests that the majority of parents of obese kids don't recognize that their child is obese.

How can you tell if your child is really overweight? Unfortunately, there isn't a foolproof measure that would tell a parent when they should be concerned about their child's weight. The Center for Disease Control (CDC) has developed growth charts that show, for each age, the percent of kids at that weight. It's difficult to use these charts but if you look online at: http://apps.nccd.cdc. gov/dnpabmi/ the CDC has a calculator that will do the work for you.

A child is technically defined as being obese if his weight is at or above the 95th percentile for his age, but the CDC charts and cut-offs are primarily intended for research purposes rather than to diagnose an individual child. For some kids, BMIs can be misleading. Since muscle is heavier than fat tissue, a muscular kid may have a BMI in the obese range even though she is not excessively fat. Whether your child meets the exact cut-off for obesity is less important than recognizing the health risks and psychological suffering that can affect all overweight kids, whether they meet the official criteria for obesity or not.

Research shows that 60 percent of overweight kids have at least one risk factor for cardiovascular disease while 20 percent of overweight kids have two risk factors. The rate of Type II diabetes (formerly called Adult Onset diabetes, but renamed because so many children developed the disease) has increased tenfold in the last decade. It's likely that the next 10 to 20 years will see an increase in kidney failure, blindness and amputations as a result of uncontrolled diabetes. Research published in *The New England Journal of Medicine* suggests that the current generation of kids will have a two- to five-year *decrease* in life expectancy because of the increase in childhood obesity. This could be the first time in our history that children will have a *shorter* life expectancy than their parents.

Todd is an example of an overweight kid who was now suffering health consequences as an adult. He told me that he couldn't remember a time when he wasn't heavy. Although his pediatrician wanted him to lose weight, his father and mother thought that he would outgrow his "baby fat." At 47, Todd still hadn't outgrown his "baby fat" and was pre-diabetic. Despite his physician's repeated warnings about diabetes and the risk of cardiovascular disease, he couldn't lose the weight necessary to get his blood glucose levels down. In desperation, he was thinking about having bariatric surgery.

Todd's parents didn't realize that there's no difference between baby fat and adult fat. Too much fat is unhealthy whether it's on a child or an adult. Researchers at the Centers for Disease Control and Prevention found that among obese toddlers, 93% of the boys and 73% of the girls became obese adults; they didn't outgrow their baby fat, it just became adult fat. An English study suggests that if obesity is established before age 11, it's more difficult to lose weight later in life. If you're concerned about your child's weight the time to act is NOW. It's going to get harder, not easier, to help your child get to a healthy weight.

## Stigma, Discrimination and Self-esteem

If your child is overweight he might not suffer the health consequences until he's older but it's likely that he's suffering the psychological consequences right now. Overweight kids feel ashamed of their bodies. This shame lowers their self-esteem and psychological well being with far-reaching consequences. In addition to feeling bad about themselves, schoolwork, after-school activities, and relations with other kids suffer. It's almost impossible for your child to escape the social discrimination and stigma associated with obesity.

Discrimination against fat people has been documented in schools, the workplace, hospitals and doctor's offices, as well as in countless daily social interactions. With laws protecting the rights of the disabled and ethnic and sexual minorities, it seems that prejudice against the overweight is the last socially acceptable form of discrimination. While no one would justify making a racist comment by claiming that it "was for his own good," many times it is perfectly acceptable to make a negative comment about someone's weight "for his own good." How many times has your child heard "helpful" (but humiliating) comments about her weight?

Stigma and discrimination against overweight people isn't limited to adults; it occurs in all age groups. Prejudice against overweight kids has been documented in kindergarten or even earlier. One study of six-year-olds found that an overweight child was described as lazy, dirty, stupid and ugly. This weight discrimination continues throughout childhood and adolescence. Another study found that almost all obese adolescent girls reported being verbally abused by their classmates. Researchers found that college students rated embezzlers, cocaine users, and shoplifters as better marriage partners than an obese person. Kids can be cruel:

- Amber's mom described seven-year-old Amber's emotional pain when she wasn't invited to a classmate's birthday party. Amber overheard one of her classmates saying that she didn't want any fat kids at the party.
- Tanya, an eighth grader, was humiliated when she was on the staircase between classes. A boy following her up the stairs made loud oinking noises followed by his imitation of a hog call.
- Two kids on the school bus called Josh, an overweight fourth grader in a class for gifted kids, a "fat pig" and "faggot."

Often overweight kids are too embarrassed to tell their parents about the humiliation they experience. Even if you haven't heard your child complain that he's been teased about his weight, you shouldn't assume that he has been spared. While the list of possible humiliations an overweight kid can suffer is endless, here are a few of the most common examples:

- Being the butt of jokes or called names;
- Being pushed, tripped, or elbowed;
- Hearing comments made to others about his appearance;
- Receiving hostile or threatening phone calls, texts, or emails;
- Being excluded from social activities;
- Being ignored in group situations;
- Having personal property damaged or stolen;
- Being hit or physically assaulted; and
- Being the subject of unflattering rumors.

Unfortunately, hurtful comments aren't just limited to cruel classmates. Often teachers, doctors, or even family members will make "helpful" or "humorous" comments with the expectation that this will encourage the child to lose weight. Of course, when the child is already feeling self-conscious about his weight, any comment that draws attention to it is hurtful and not likely to motivate a child to lose weight.

Overweight kids tend to withdraw from social interactions, spend more time in sedentary activities, become increasingly isolated, and often turn to food for nurturance. Confronted with continued rejection, is it any wonder that a child might use food to feel better? There's evidence that being teased results in significant increases in binge eating. For example, Jenny was the "fat kid" throughout her childhood and adolescence. In elementary school her classmates teased her almost every day. In P.E. classes, when it was time to choose up teams for softball, volleyball or any other sport, Jenny was the last one chosen. In high school she avoided going to dances because she knew she wouldn't be asked to dance. At family get-togethers her uncle often made "humorous" comments about her weight. Over the years, Jenny became more withdrawn and spent much of her free time by herself, watching TV while consoling herself with large quantities of food.

If your child experiences this type of discrimination, imagine the emotional consequences. Even if you do your best to be supportive at home it's unlikely that you'll be able to compensate for all the rejection and humiliation he or she receives. While you are helping your child to lose weight, what can you do to minimize this suffering?

## Encourage Socializing

One partial solution was suggested by a study from the State University of New York at Buffalo. The results showed that, for nine- to eleven-year-old children, having friends and socializing can be a substitute for eating. If you sense that your child is starting to withdraw or that she has fewer friends, try to encourage more social contacts. Get your child involved in Boy Scouts, Girl Scouts or other after-school activity. If necessary, you can arrange play dates or organize fun activities that include other children. Helping your child to be social will decrease teasing and minimize solitary, mindless TV viewing and eating.

## Listen

When a child has been teased about his weight he may just want a sympathetic ear, rather than suggestions on how to cope. Before you provide advice, listen carefully. Don't say anything until your child fully describes what happened. When he's finished, communicate your understanding. Often this can be as simple as just maintaining eye contact and nodding sympathetically.

You can explain that teasing is usually the result of insecurity on the part of the person doing the teasing. To make himself feel better, the teaser needs to find someone else to put down. Often the teaser is trying to join the popular group in school. He thinks that, by making fun of you he will look more confident and self-assured so the popular kids will like him. The kid doing the teasing should be pitied rather than feared.

## Inoculate Your Child

You can't follow your child to school and all the other places where she's likely to be teased. What you can do is "inoculate" your child so that negative comments from others have minimal impact and when necessary, she can respond to maintain her dignity.

If it seems that your child is looking for help in responding to weight-related taunts, you can suggest:

- Don't look embarrassed or intimidated, maintain your composure and be confident.
- Don't give the bully the pleasure of responding, fighting back, or showing any emotion. Eventually, the bully will get bored and find something else to do.
- Tell an adult you can trust — a parent, teacher, or coach who doesn't approve of bullying. This isn't tattling, but rather, you are showing that you can't be intimidated.
- If a trusted adult or family member is doing the teasing, let them know that it is hurtful and doesn't help you to lose weight.

# Chapter 3 - Winning the Battle
# Without Losing the War

Parents, especially parents of girls, walk a very narrow tightrope. If you're reading this book you're concerned about your child's weight and want to do everything possible to encourage healthy eating and exercise habits, but you may also be aware of the dangers of eating disorders. Almost all children and teens that become anorexic or bulimic report a history of dieting to lose weight. Often they report that a well-meaning adult, sometimes a parent or possibly a teacher, pediatrician, coach, or relative, commented on their weight and suggested that they go on a diet. The child may have had some success losing weight and enjoyed the compliments she received. Sometimes the dieting doesn't stop with a healthy weight loss but snowballs out of control, resulting in anorexia nervosa.

Anorexia is the most deadly psychiatric diagnosis, with as many as 20 percent of anorexics dying from complications of the disorder. Many more anorexics don't die but live their lives gravely disabled. They suffer the effects of malnutrition and lead lives greatly constricted by a distorted body image and the need to avoid gaining weight. There are many possible causes of anorexia and most girls who go on diets don't become anorexic, yet, considering the risks, parents need to be careful when discussing weight with their children.

When Kelly was 11 she became concerned about her "poochy" stomach so she stopped eating bread and other starchy food. Her parents had been concerned about her weight so they were pleased that Kelly was dieting and had become health conscious. Over the next few months, however, they became concerned as Kelly increased the number of foods that were off limits and her weight decreased sharply. She also developed some strange eating habits, like only eating foods in certain combinations or in a particular order.

Kelly was 20 years old when she was referred to me. She weighed 105 pounds and was so afraid of eating that her hand would shake when she picked up a fork with food on it. Although she knew that her extreme dieting made her tired and frequently dizzy, she couldn't force herself to eat. Ten months later she moved to a new town and I lost track of her. Before the move she had made significant progress and had gained some weight, but still saw herself as fat and wasn't completely comfortable eating. I wonder what would have been different if her parents had sought professional help earlier.

While an emphasis on dieting and weight causes some young people to become anorexic, many more try to diet but don't succeed in losing weight. It takes incredible self-discipline to overcome the body's intense signals when it's being malnourished. When confronted with hunger pangs, lightheadedness, and the fatigue that comes with starvation, most dieting children relent and eat, frequently huge quantities of foods that had been forbidden on their diet. Since they're not losing weight, dieting kids may become increasingly frantic and resort to more desperate measures. Most often it's self-induced vomiting, but sometimes it's laxative abuse or over-exercising. When this becomes a pattern, it's classified as bulimia nervosa, a disorder that is less fatal than anorexia nervosa, but still results in serious medical and psychological complications.

Ann R. was a single, 25-year-old Japanese-American woman who worked for a major pharmaceutical firm as a researcher. She consulted me when she broke up with her long-term boyfriend after he announced that he was bisexual. In addition to coming to terms with the painful break-up, Anne was concerned that her weight had shot up to 160 pounds (BMI = 29.2) and her bulimia had gotten worse.

Ann's mother was overweight, and, trying to prevent Ann from becoming too heavy, Mrs. R. put Ann on a diet at age eight. Throughout high school and college Ann tried many diets, Nutrisystem, Jenny Craig, and in desperation, abused laxatives and resorted to making herself vomit. When I first saw her she was throwing up almost every day. After each episode, Ann would feel shame and disgust and vow that next time she would stick to her diet.

One of the many negative consequences of bulimia is that, after a binge-purge episode, the bulimic usually intensifies her efforts to diet and becomes more extreme in avoiding the "bad" foods forbidden by her diet. Of course, this rarely works, and instead is just making another binge-purge episode more likely. Fortunately for Ann, we were able to stop the binge-purge cycle. With counseling she was able to give up dieting and find a more realistic method of regulating her eating. Gradually she accepted the idea that at five feet, three inches tall she was never going to look like a model, but she was still smart and cute and would find another boyfriend.

Parents of anorexic children usually notice when their child greatly restricts her eating and loses weight. Often they start with excuses for not eating — "I ate at my friend's house," or "I had a big snack, so I'm not hungry," but eventually they just become defiant in refusing to eat as they lose weight. On the other hand, parents of bulimic children may not see any signs of the eating disorder. Typically bulimics are embarrassed about their binge-purge behaviors and go to great lengths to avoid detection, but parents may notice that their child is preoccupied with weight and dieting. Sometimes the child becomes more secretive and food or money is missing. If you suspect that your child might be anorexic or bulimic, it's important that you educate yourself about eating disorders and seek professional help. Early intervention increases the likelihood that treatment will be successful. A good place to start is www.anad.org.

Many teens, even if they don't have an eating disorder will resort to unhealthy means to control their weight. Some teens take up smoking, use diet pills or ADHD medications like Adderall or Ritalin to suppress their appetite. These methods are harmful and ultimately unsuccessful.

As a parent, you don't want your child to suffer the health and psychological consequences of obesity, but if you make them feel miserable about being fat, or scare them with horror stories about the effects of gaining weight you could lay the groundwork for an eating disorder. Your task is to help your child win the obesity battle without losing the eating disorders war. The 10 Steps to a healthy weight will show you how do it.

# Chapter 4 – Looking In the Mirror

Before you can help your child lose weight, you'll need to examine your thinking about obesity. Many widely held beliefs would interfere with your attempts to help your child, so let's look at your assumptions about weight gain to see if you should change your thinking. It will help to understand the psychology of weight bias and obesity stigma – why is it viewed so negatively? Then we'll examine the role parents play in determining their child's weight. You may be relieved to find that it's not all your fault!

## Obesity As a Moral Defect

It's unfortunate that being overweight is not usually seen as a medical problem or even a behavioral challenge. If you listen carefully, it often seems that obesity is thought of as a moral problem. Fat people are "guilty" if they eat a calorie-rich food that is "illegal," they are "lazy" if they don't exercise, and "weak-willed" if they can't stick to their diet. Thinking about obesity in these morally laden terms results in a tremendous stigma associated with being overweight. After all, if someone is guilty, lazy, and weak-willed, they don't deserve the same respect and privileges that morally superior people of a normal weight enjoy.

Tim and Marilyn had heard me speak at a PTA meeting and were in my office to discuss Matt, their fifth grader. Matt's weight put his BMI in the 90th percentile for kids his age. When I asked the parents to tell me about Matt, Tim used the term "lazy" to describe his son. I followed up and asked Tim to explain.

"When the other kids are out playing ball, riding bikes, or just goofing around, Matt is in his room watching TV or playing games on the computer. We've tried to get him to stop, but usually he's eating something too. He gets into the chips, and sometimes we've caught him sneaking cookies into his room. Who knows what he spends his lunch money on?"

I probed a little further, asking, "Is he lazy in other ways? Does he do his homework? Help with chores? Watch his little brother when you ask him to?"

Marilyn came to her son's defense. She said, "Sometimes we have to nag him to do his chores, but he's no worse than any other kid his age. He's very good about schoolwork and he's reliable when watching his brother."

I suggested that the word "lazy" is just a description of some behaviors, a label we attach to these behaviors. Calling someone lazy doesn't really explain why a kid (or an adult, for that matter) behaves the way he does. We should look at what else is going on in the child's life to really understand why he does what he does.

Tim acknowledged that Marilyn was right about the homework and chores. He understood that Matt really wasn't lazy; he had always been a shy kid and wasn't very coordinated, so he didn't enjoy sports and felt awkward around some of his classmates. When Tim understood his son's difficulties, he felt closer to him. Tim suggested that the two of them could ride bikes together on weekends and perhaps they could invite one of the neighborhood kids to come along.

Once we give up the idea that obesity is a result of laziness, a weak will or some other kind of moral defect, it's possible to view obesity as a problem that, with some effort, can be addressed. It also helps to understand your feelings about your child's weight. If you view extra pounds as evidence of laziness or lack of will power, your child will sense your disappointment and feel badly. Guilt and shame rarely inspire a child to lose weight. Instead, it usually results in withdrawal and frequently, in sneaky behavior regarding food and eating. Any attempt to help your child is likely to backfire if she knows that you are angry, or even just disappointed with her.

If you have negative feelings it will make it difficult for your child to comply with any suggestions you offer. Eating can become a battleground where you and she engage in a mutually destructive fight, leaving everyone unhappy and your child still overweight. Instead, try to view your child's weight as a problem that needs to be resolved rather than as a weakness in your child's character.

## Is Obesity a Result of Bad Parenting?

Some parents may not see their child's obesity as a character problem, but still communicate their disappointment because they are embarrassed by their child's weight. When you are in public settings with your child, do you feel that your child reflects badly on you? Are you concerned that other people will think that you are an inadequate parent because you let your child get heavy?

Susan and Charles L. were the parents of Julia, a bright, energetic, overweight 12-year-old. When Susan came home from PTA meetings, teacher conferences, or even if she ran into a neighbor when she and Julia were shopping at the mall, Susan was embarrassed because of Julia's weight. Usually she increased her efforts to put Julia on a diet. For the next few days Susan would be carefully monitoring Julia's eating and issuing directives on what to eat and what was forbidden. Julia felt bad because she sensed her mother's embarrassment, but Julia's unhappiness only propelled her to eat more, not less.

It may help to recognize that we live in an environment that makes gaining weight effortless. Think about all the people your child sees eating, all the food commercials on TV, the restaurants she sees when driving by, the vending machines, and the well-stocked pantries and refrigerators at home. Every day your child will encounter thousands of food cues increasing the urge to eat. Regardless of what their parents may do or say, even iron-willed kids would have difficulty ignoring these cues. It would be a lot easier to stay slim if there weren't so many cues temping us to eat and so many opportunities to give in. With the 10 Steps you'll be able to create an environment that reduces eating opportunities while making physical activity more likely.

## Is Obesity a Result of Good Parenting?

If you have had your own struggles with weight, you may want to insure that your child doesn't have the same unpleasant experiences you've had. If you're currently overweight, you correctly recognize that it's easier to prevent obesity in childhood instead of trying to lose weight as an adult. Elaine, a 43-year-old mother, recalled her adolescent struggles with weight and diets that resulted in a several-year bout of bulimia. She was determined that Stacy, her nine-year-old daughter, would be spared even though Stacy had inherited Elaine's large frame.

Elaine was a sensitive mom, and unlike Mrs. S. (Julie's mom described in Chapter 1), Elaine was not dictatorial. Rather, Elaine had a heart-to-heart talk with her daughter. She described her own struggles with weight and patiently explained to Stacy why she shouldn't eat junk foods or high calorie snacks. When Elaine found Stacy eating one of the prohibited foods Elaine kept her cool, and carefully explained again why Stacy should avoid these foods. It didn't help; Stacy still gained weight even though she felt guilty for disappointing her mother.

All the understanding and sincere heart-to-heart talks might bring you closer to your overweight child, but probably won't result in weight loss. Talking, however heartfelt and well intentioned, isn't enough. You'll need a more active approach to helping your child. The 10 Steps are designed to do just that.

## How Do You Talk to Your Child About Weight?

Although the 10 Steps will have you actively participating rather than just telling your child what to do, there will be times when you'll need to discuss the changes you are making. When you are having these discussions it's important that you don't communicate anger, frustration, shame, or embarrassment. Start by examining your deepest feelings about your child's weight. Ask yourself:

- Are you embarrassed when you and your child are with slender kids and their parents?
- Are you afraid that people are going to think that you're an inadequate parent because you've got an overweight child?
- If you're overweight too, are you concerned that your child's weight will draw attention to your struggles with weight?

If you harbor these feelings, it's quite likely that your child will sense your uneasiness and feel bad for causing your discomfort. It may seem paradoxical, but this will only make it harder for your child to lose weight.

In order to help your child, you'll have to adopt an emotionally neutral, problem-solving attitude about his weight. If you find this hard to do, consider how you would feel if your child was blind. It might be awkward if he stumbled in public, but you'd be sympathetic and try to shield him from any embarrassment. You'd be supportive and work with him to help him cope with the challenges his disability presents. You certainly wouldn't blame him for being blind even if the blindness resulted from an accident caused by his carelessness. The same attitude will help with your overweight child. Even if he is partially responsible for his weight gain, you'll need to be supportive, not critical, to help him develop healthy eating and exercise habits. Here are some guidelines for communicating with your child about her eating and weight:

- Expect frustration —— despite your best efforts, a change in habit doesn't happen overnight.
- If you find yourself getting angry with your overweight child call a timeout. Yelling or name calling will undermine all your efforts.
- Don't compare your child with siblings or other kids.
- With young children, encourage them to eat healthy foods but let them decide how much to eat.
- With teens, don't bring up the topic of their weight, but when they raise the issue or just make a comment about their weight, ask, "What can I do to help?"
- Don't criticize unhealthy behaviors but do praise healthy ones.

- Defend your child when adults tease or make "helpful" or "humorous" comments about his weight.

# Part II – 10 Steps to a Healthy Weight

The 10 Steps are useful for all overweight kids, but not all kids and families have the same challenges. You may find some of the steps less relevant for your circumstances, and how you implement each step will depend in part on the specifics of your household and on your child's age. In addition to suggesting specific methods for each step, I've tried to provide a rationale for the step based on research and clinical experience. Understanding the rationale will help you tailor the implementation to your specific situation.

When preschool children are at home, a direct approach is often easiest – you tell your child what you expect him to do and provide clear guidelines for how to do it. When your child is in nursery school, daycare, or off to kindergarten, telling her what to do becomes less effective. You don't have any control over their environment when they're at school or their friends' houses. For pre-teens and teenagers, giving directions may not work and often telling them what to do can precipitate rebelliousness or efforts to sneak food. They may just refuse to comply, or like Julie, do what they want when you're not around. Keep in mind that *telling a child what to do is only one way, and often not the best way, of influencing her behavior.*

Although the results may not be immediate, parents can influence their child's behavior, even a rebellious adolescent's behavior with three other strategies:

1. Alter the environment —— although a school-aged child may spend most of his waking hours away from the home, you still can change the household

environment to make desirable behaviors more likely.

2. Model desirable behavior —— even teens who think that their parents are complete geeks still look to their parents for guidance, although they might never admit it.

3. Reward good behavior —— often a simple, age-appropriate comment can increase the chances that the behavior will be repeated. Just make sure that the praise is sincere and expressed in a way that sounds natural.

Don't get discouraged or frustrated if you don't see immediate results. Be persistent, changing habits takes time.

# Step 1: Prompt, Don't Push — Retreat Gracefully and Try Again Another Day

Does it seem like getting your kids to try new foods is an ongoing struggle? Many kids are willing to try almost any dessert, but refuse foods that aren't sweet. It may help to know that your child's preference for sweet foods isn't just stubbornness — your child is just following patterns established by our prehistoric ancestors.

Humans are born liking sweet foods, everything else we have to learn to like. Our innate preference for sweet tastes may be a remnant from our prehistoric ancestors' struggle to survive. Poisonous substances rarely taste sweet so our ancestors who ate sweet foods were more likely to survive, those who ate bitter or sour substances were more likely to be poisoned. Now, countless generations later, your kids prefer sweet tastes and routinely refuse anything that has a strong flavor like onions, garlic, or bitter vegetables. The task for you as a parent is to help your child overcome her reluctance to try new foods that aren't sweet.

## The Breastfeeding Advantage

If your child was breastfed, she may have a head start in learning to like new foods. One review of nine studies with almost 70,000 participants found that breastfed children were less likely to be overweight. It's not clear why breastfeeding decreases the likelihood of childhood obesity. It's possible that the composition of breast milk may contain substances that have a positive effect on your baby's metabolism, but it's also likely that babies learn to stop eating when they're full if they've been breastfed.

When an infant is bottle-fed, the parent doing the feeding determines how much formula the infant should take. You look at the bottle and can see how much formula your child has consumed. You give him more or less until you think he's had enough. When the infant is breastfed, it's more difficult for a parent to know how much he's consumed. When he has had enough the nipple just slips from his mouth. Baby decides how much he needs and stops when he's satisfied. He's learning to regulate his eating based on his biological needs rather than having someone else do it for him.

Breastfeeding may also help a child enjoy a balanced diet when he's older. There's some evidence that it may be easier for infants who have been breastfed to try new foods. If your infant is bottle-fed he will experience the same taste day after day. On the other hand, if Mom breast-feeds her baby, he will be exposed to different tastes depending on what Mom had to eat that day. When he becomes a toddler, there might be less reluctance to try new foods.

### Fighting Over Vegetables

It's easy to get frustrated if your child fights you when you try to introduce a new food. You're concerned about your child's health so you're trying to help him eat a balanced diet. You are the adult who is in control, but yet your toddler or preschooler is ignoring your good intentions and sincere efforts. Sometimes it seems that he enjoys your frustration.

Marie was confronted with this dilemma. She'd prepare a balanced meal that included a vegetable dish, which her daughter, Samantha, routinely refused. Marie tried all the usual strategies. When Samantha was a toddler, Marie tried to make a game of eating vegetables.

She'd say, "Open up, here's a train coming into the station." This was accompanied by Marie's attempt to make engine chugging noises as the vegetable-laden fork approached her daughter's mouth. Usually the train got derailed before it ever got to the station.

When Samantha was a preschooler, Marie offered the veggies and pleaded, "Just try a little, you'll like it." Samantha wouldn't and didn't. Marie became impatient when she felt that Samantha enjoyed frustrating her. Once, when Marie wasn't having a good day, she tried to force Samantha's mouth open to insert the vegetables. This didn't work either.

As Samantha got older, Marie's strategies evolved. When Samantha joined a soccer team, Marie told her she'd need to eat her vegetables to get strong so she could be a better player. When Samantha started noticing boys, Marie reminded her that vegetables didn't have a lot of calories. If she ate her vegetables she would stay thin and be more attractive to boys. Despite Samantha's interest in soccer and boys, Marie's arguments were rarely persuasive.

Sometimes Marie resorted to bribery: "You can't have dessert until you've finished your vegetables." Samantha rarely complied. Instead, she'd sacrifice dessert. If she really wanted the dessert, Samantha would wait until dinner was over and her parents were watching TV. Then she'd go back into the kitchen and help herself to the dessert she'd missed. Regardless of Marie's efforts, Samantha rarely ate her vegetables.

How can you avoid this ongoing battle? Several recent books advocate sneaking pureed vegetables into recipes for foods that children enjoy. While this strategy offers short-term benefits, you'll want your kids to eat vegetables when you're not preparing special dishes for them. Rather than relying on "covert operations" in the kitchen, it may help to recognize that, at least initially, a child's reluctance to try new foods is not a result of stubbornness or defiance. With infants and toddlers you are challenging thousands of years of evolution that have programmed your child to resist. Try to avoid getting into a battle of wills. Instead, be patient. It may take many repetitions, perhaps ten, twelve or more, for a child to become comfortable with a novel taste.

Whatever you do, you don't want to make this process more difficult by confounding eating with your child's drive for independence. Regardless of age, your son or daughter will be striving to become more independent. A preschooler will want to tie his own shoes; a ten-year-old will want to stay up later; while a teen will argue about the curfew you've imposed. It's natural for children to strive to be free of parental control, but we want to prevent food choice from becoming a battleground in your child's struggle for independence.

On the other hand, you do want your child to try new foods, and if you are completely passive, he might not try broccoli until he's in his 40's, so the best strategy is to introduce the food and briefly encourage your child to try it. Start with sweet vegetables like carrots or peas; save the asparagus for later. If he refuses, don't offer a different food — your child isn't going to starve if he misses part of a meal. Don't get angry and avoid lengthy explanations, pleading, or coercing. Instead, if your child refuses, just try again next week. If many repetitions aren't working, consider the following:

- Use a different recipe to introduce the new food. Sometimes a simple change, like adding melted cheese to a vegetable dish or using different spices, is enough to entice the child to try the new food.

- Without a lot of discussion, make sure your child sees that you are enjoying the new food. When children are very young they enjoy pretending to be Mommy or Daddy. When they get a little older, they may not deliberately imitate their parents, but parents still have a powerful impact on their behavior. Find some vegetable dishes that you enjoy and let your kids see you eat them with enthusiasm.
- Have your child help you prepare the new food. For younger children, helping Mom or Dad prepare the vegetable can be part of getting ready for a special event like a family celebration or Thanksgiving dinner. After spending an afternoon in the kitchen cooking the new dish, it's less likely that your child will refuse to try it.
- Help your child plant a vegetable garden and have her help pick and prepare the vegetables she's grown.

One frequently used technique that you should *avoid* is making dessert a reward for eating the new food. I have had personal experience with this approach. Like Samantha, my parents often told me, "You can't have dessert (usually ice cream) until you've finished your vegetables." The implicit message being communicated is that ice cream is more desirable than vegetables. Although it may seem that ice cream is intrinsically more desirable than vegetables, I know several people who prefer well-prepared vegetables to ice cream. Believe it or not, one friend rarely eats ice cream but gets excited about Brussels sprouts! The goal for parents is to make eating vegetables a rewarding experience rather than something that requires a bribe.

## Action Plan:

1. The new vegetable(s) I will introduce are _____
   _____ and _____.

2. I will prepare one of these vegetables approximately
   every ___ days, and let my child see me enjoy eating
   it.

3. After ___ refusals, I will alter the recipe and try
   again.

4. If my child still refuses on _____ (date), I will
   have him help to prepare one of these vegetable
   dishes.

## Step 2: Structure Eating Around Three Sit-down Meals and One or Two Planned Snacks

Unfortunately, family dinners seem to be a disappearing ritual. Regular meals provide structure for the child's eating. Eating together also offers parents the opportunity to model good eating behaviors. Family dinners should be a pleasant experience with no distractions. If you're in the habit of having the television on while eating, it may feel strange to turn it off, but the benefits are worth the awkwardness of the temporary adjustment period.

Once you turn off the TV and get the kids to stop texting while at the table, family dinners can be a relaxing time for you to find out what's going on in their lives. Even if you encounter initial resistance, or a sullen refusal to respond with anything more than a grunt or "fine" in response to your attempts to foster communication, don't give up, it's still worth doing. Make the dinner experience pleasant so save lectures about bad grades, chores that have been ignored, or misbehavior for some other time when you're not eating.

Some young people avoid meals because they are dieting. For example, Holly, a 20-year-old college student, consulted me because her bulimia had gotten out of control. When I asked her to keep track of her eating, she, like most bulimics, didn't want to write down what she'd been eating. She acknowledged that it was difficult to write everything down because it would make her feel guilty about how much she ate. Reluctantly, she agreed to keep track of her eating using the forms I provided.

We reviewed her eating records the following week. I was amazed to find that she rarely had a meal because she "was on a diet." Almost all of her eating was comprised of intermittent snacking. During a typical day she didn't have breakfast. When I suggested that she eat breakfast she said, "Why should I eat breakfast when I'm not hungry? I don't even like cereal." Of course, she would snack on the way to class, have a burrito from the cafeteria after class, chips from the vending machine later in the afternoon, a slice of the pizza that her friend had ordered, and so on.

Holly thought she could lose weight by skipping meals. She ignored the typical mealtimes (breakfast at 7:30, lunch at noon, for example). She frequently felt hungry but learned to ignore the hunger sensations. As a result, Holly didn't have any of the physiological signals that would help her know when to eat and when she didn't need to eat. So she lacked both the internal (hunger) and external (meal times) guidelines to regulate her eating. Holly's eating became disorganized, and when she did eat, she made poor choices. Instead of balanced meals she ate high calorie snack foods. Since she had skipped meals she was very hungry so, once she did start to eat, it was hard to stop and she frequently overate. Afterwards she felt horrible for "going off the diet," so she made herself throw up.

I had Holly consult a dietitian who developed a meal plan that provided structure for her eating. That, combined with the counseling to address some of Holly's psychological issues, resulted in a marked decrease in bingeing and she lost, rather than gained, a few pounds by having regular meals and snacks.

It's not likely that your child's eating is as chaotic as Holly's was but it's never too early to establish a pattern of regular meals and snacks. Even if it takes some rearranging of your own schedule, it's important to provide structure to your child's eating so that he develops his own internal guidelines for eating.

You have some control over your child's eating at home but structuring your child's eating in school is more difficult. Although you can't have lunch with your child in school, you should be aware of what she is eating. If you prepare the lunch, check occasionally to be sure that she's actually eating what you've made. If your child eats lunch in the school cafeteria, keep track of the school's menu (frequently it's available online) and, if you have concerns, let the principal know or, perhaps, bring it up at a PTA meeting.

Once children reach their teens they may be drawn into after school activities, sports practice, or just hanging-out with friends so that they're not home at dinnertime. Requiring attendance at dinnertime can be fighting an uphill battle. Instead, try to find one, two or more nights each week when there aren't competing activities and establish a family dinner night routine. Even if it requires rearranging schedules, it's worth the effort. Research suggests that when families eat together kids eat more fruits and vegetables and less fried foods. Teens who eat with their families are less likely to get involved in risky behaviors. Although it isn't necessary to use your finest china, it is necessary to relax, turn off iPods, cell phones, and television, and talk rather than text during dinner.

## Mom Was Right About Breakfast

Did your mother ever tell you, "Breakfast is the most important meal?" She was right but you may be in the habit of skipping it because you're "not hungry" or "too busy" and think that you're saving calories by not eating breakfast. In my work with obese and bulimic clients, I frequently hear objections when I suggest that they start eating breakfast. Like Holly, Diana, a 22-year-old college student, didn't eat breakfast. She told me, "I'm not even hungry in the morning. Why should I have 300 calories that I don't need and don't want?"

It was difficult to persuade her to try having a low-calorie, high-fiber cereal with skim milk and a slice of cheese (the milk and cheese provide protein, which will delay hunger pangs). I pointed out that although it may seem paradoxical, eating breakfast is a useful weight loss strategy. One study of over 16,000 people showed that the thinnest people surveyed had hot cereal for breakfast, followed by cold cereal eaters. The heaviest people were breakfast skippers.

I don't know what your experience has been but I find that if I miss a meal I'm ravenously hungry when I finally do eat. As a result, I eat too fast and frequently overeat. If your child skips breakfast she may have a similar experience. It's likely that she'll be starving by the time she finally does eat. Once she starts eating she'll find it difficult to pace her eating, so it's likely that she'll gobble her food quickly. She'll eat a lot of food in a short time period before she starts to feel sated. In addition to eating more than she needs, she might have the uncomfortable sense that her eating is out of control, which could increase her fear of gaining weight.

Eating breakfast will help your child regulate her food consumption and reduce the chance that she'll overeat later in the day. Diana reluctantly acknowledged that, often when she didn't eat breakfast, she had a hard time controlling her eating in the afternoon and continued overeating at night. Once she started having breakfast she wasn't as hungry later in the day so that when she did eat, it didn't feel like an uncontrolled binge.

You might recognize the importance of breakfast but feel that you can't fit it into your schedule. For many families, mornings are particularly hectic. It may be difficult getting your kids up and ready for school and then getting yourself and your spouse out the door on time. With so much going on in the morning, you're probably reluctant to add any new demands to your schedule. The simple solution to this problem is having everyone wake-up 15 minutes earlier and have the cereal and drinks ready to go. If the cereal is out, and milk and cheese close at hand, how difficult would it be to have the kids eat breakfast? Now is the time to start.

## Snacks and Treats

For many kids, after school snacks contribute a significant number of unnecessary calories. If your child has lunch in school at noon, it's unrealistic to expect him to go until dinner at 6:30 or 7:00 without eating something in between. As a rule it's best to have your kids eat every four hours. This will help keep their blood sugar levels stable and prevent them from getting too hungry. What should they eat when they get home from school? Rather than providing the traditional milk and cookies, consider some less sweet alternatives. Apples or other fruit, cheese, air-popped popcorn, baked chips, and nuts are healthy alternatives.

I think it's helpful to make a distinction between snacks and treats. A snack is something you eat in-between meals to satisfy your physical hunger. In contrast, a treat like ice cream, cookies, or candy is a food you eat purely for enjoyment. You shouldn't think of treats as bad and try to forbid them, but instead accept them as one of life's pleasures to be enjoyed in moderation. It's best to save treats for special occasions or to use as desserts. There's evidence suggesting that, when a high calorie treat is consumed after dinner, when you're no longer hungry, the future cravings for that food decrease, so save the sweet goodies for dessert. Don't offer them when your kids are hungry after school.

Christine is the proud mother of three slender young women in their twenties. None of the three has a "sweet tooth" nor are they especially fond of chocolates or other desserts. When I asked Christine how she was able to avoid the downfall of so many young girls, she thought for a while and recalled that when her daughters were in school, there were no cookies or sweet snacks in the house. She told me, "When the girls came home from school they were hungry so I gave them apple slices or oranges to eat. Since they weren't accustomed to having cookies they didn't complain and happily ate the fruit for their snack. If they were at a friend's house they might have had a cookie, and on special occasions they baked cookies with their grandmother, but they rarely had them in our house."

If your kids haven't started school yet, it's best not to keep sweets in the house. If you or your spouse feels the need to have a cookie, go to a bakery, buy one and really enjoy the experience, but don't keep them in the house to use for snacking. If your kids already are in the habit of having cookies when they come home from school, don't despair. You can wean them off this habit or at least minimize the damage.

If you must have cookies or other sugary treats in the house, buy them in single serving packs. It may be less expensive to buy the large economy size but this encourages overeating. On the other hand, if your child knows that he is entitled to one small pack, and that you've been keeping track of the number being consumed, you will reduce the tendency to have seconds (and thirds). In addition to the sweet snack, provide a healthier alternative like fruit, nuts, or cheese slices. Nuts are especially valuable because the feeling of satiation they provide lasts longer than other snacks so there will be less need for additional eating as the afternoon wears on. When your child becomes accustomed to having the healthy foods along with the cookies, see if you can't reduce and possibly eliminate the cookies from the afternoon snack.

## Action Plan:

1. I will serve _____ for breakfast at _____ a.m. on weekdays and at _____ a.m. on weekends.

2. I will tell the kids that on _____ (specify days of the week) we will be having dinner together as a family at _____ p.m. so they shouldn't plan other activities for that time.

3. I will offer _____ or _____ as healthy afternoon snacks.

4. If my children are in the habit of having cookies or other high-calorie treats when they come home from school, I will provide single serving packages along with the healthier snacks.

# Step 3: Don't Put Your Child on a Diet — Instead Encourage Healthy Eating

When most adults want to lose weight they go on a diet. It rarely works, but this is the commonly accepted strategy for weight loss. It's understandable, then, that when adults want their children to lose weight, they put the kids on a diet too. Several carefully controlled studies have demonstrated that dieting usually results in weight GAIN for children.

When parents put their kid on a diet they are attempting to control their child's eating. One thorough review of 22 studies found that excessive parental control of eating increases their kids' liking for the foods that are forbidden. Dieting disrupts the child's natural self-regulation. Your child will depend on the diet rules —— what to eat and what not to eat —— that you've imposed. These external rules cause the child to UNLEARN the natural processes that she should use to determine when and how much to eat.

In addition to gaining weight, childhood dieting can stigmatize your child and lower his self-esteem. When all his friends are having a Slurpee, how will he feel if he has to explain to them that he can't have one because he's on a diet? To avoid being left out he'll probably relent and have the forbidden food, but then feel guilty because he didn't follow his diet. In addition to feeling guilty, he may feel that he needs to lie to you about the Slurpee because he doesn't want to disappoint you. Unfortunately, the inevitable frustration with failed dieting can contribute to the development of an eating disorder. Almost all bulimics describe a lengthy history of dieting failures before they began their self-destructive behaviors.

If your child is overweight, banish the word "diet" from your vocabulary. From now on, think in terms of developing healthy eating habits rather than dieting. To be a healthy eater we need to consider what your child eats and how he eats it.

## What to Eat

For younger children, it's helpful to describe foods in terms of traffic lights: Green, Yellow and Red. Older kids might not be impressed with the traffic light categories but the same principles still apply. Kids should eat plenty of Green foods like fruits, vegetables, fish, whole grains, and many dairy products. Green foods will give your kids a lot of nutrition for fewer calories. One study of children between five and eighteen years old found that eating more fruit and vegetables was associated with less likelihood of being overweight. Although the evidence isn't conclusive, it's thought that the fiber in fruits and vegetables may help prevent obesity. Fiber doesn't have many calories and stays in the stomach longer, increasing the time before your child gets hungry again. The calcium found in dairy products may also help prevent obesity so dairy products, without added sweeteners, are also Green foods.

Yellow foods, like Green foods, provide a lot of nutrition but unlike Green foods, Yellow foods are high in calories so they should be consumed in moderation. Potatoes (but not French fries), low-fat cheese, lean meat, high fiber breads and cereals, rice, nuts, and poultry are Yellow foods.

Red foods are high in calories and have little or no nutritional value. Perhaps the reddest of Red foods are sodas and other sugary drinks. A 12-ounce can of Coke has 145 calories, has no nutritional value, and doesn't do anything to satisfy hunger. Although they are marketed as healthy, sports drinks (they usually have an "ade" in their name) are also filled with empty calories. There is some evidence that sugar in liquids causes more weight gain than sugar in other forms. One recent study found that kids who had two sodas a day were three times as likely to be overweight, so do you really want to triple the likelihood that your kids will be obese? Instead of sugary drinks, consider offering water or, if you're not concerned about the chemicals, buy diet sodas. Other Red foods include most desserts and many snack foods. Fried chicken, bacon, and French fries are examples of Red foods that aren't desserts or snacks.

One way of cutting the calories consumed at a meal is to serve hearty portions of fruits before a meal or vegetables as a first course. Research suggests that children will eat more of the produce they like and will compensate by eating smaller amounts of the foods that are served later.

## Avoiding, But Not Forbidding Red Foods

Red foods should be avoided, but not forbidden. When you're concerned about your child's weight you don't want him adding the "empty calories" from Red foods, so you might be tempted to tell him not to eat "junk food." Unfortunately, banning any food is likely to result in increasing the attractiveness of that food, and can cause binge eating.

Remember Julie S., the third grader described earlier? Mrs. S. was very firm in establishing the foods that were forbidden to Julie. Initially, she tried to patiently explain to her daughter that eating Oreos and other high calorie treats would make her fat. Julie told her mom that she understood, and wouldn't have any more Oreos. She was able to resist for several weeks, but one day, after prolonged teasing by her brother, Julie was upset and headed for the pantry where the Oreos were kept. Once she started, she didn't stop until the whole package was finished.

Forbidding a food is an example of all-or-nothing thinking. You're not allowed ANY of the food, so when you break the rule and have one, you might as well have them all. If you've been a dieter, you're probably familiar with this phenomenon. You've successfully avoided the food but then something stressful happens, you feel an urge to console yourself with the food that you've been missing, and once you've broken the rule you think, "What the hell, I've blown my diet." and proceed to binge on the forbidden food.

This is what happened to Julie, and if you try to forbid any food or group of foods, it's what will happen with your child. Unfortunately, Mrs. S. persisted in her attempts to prohibit Oreos. She became more emphatic, harshly criticizing each of Julie's infractions, resulting in an escalating battle of wills. As Mrs. S. became more critical Julie responded by becoming more devious. When Julie was a teenager, eating forbidden food became one method she used to try to assert her independence from her parents.

Even without Mrs. S's harsh criticism, forbidding any food results in two undesirable consequences: the food becomes more desirable, and the child has less ability to control his eating when the food is available. As a general rule, when something is scarce we tend to value it highly and will go to great lengths to obtain it. When Julie couldn't have Oreos, she thought about them more often and their value increased. Now, in Julie's thinking, the pleasure she would get from eating them was exaggerated. Also, by forbidding them, Mrs. S. was taking over control of Julie's eating, rather than teaching her how to control her own eating habits.

Instead of forbidding Red foods, you can explain to your child that the attractive food is not something that we eat routinely, but rather it's an occasional treat. Whenever you can, try to find a substitute for the Red food. Even if your child is currently overweight, and the Red food is high in calories and nutritionally worthless, the goal is to help him establish internal regulation and decrease the likelihood of all-or-nothing binges.

Fast food restaurants are a dangerous "Red District" for kids. Most of the foods served at these establishments are high in fat and sugar and low in fiber. You won't find many fruits and non-starchy vegetables on their menus. On average, a child's fast food meal will have 187 calories more than a meal served at home. This adds six extra pounds each year. It's not surprising that children who eat at fast food restaurants several times a week have higher BMIs than kids who eat there once a week or less. Minimizing, but not forbidding, meals at fast food restaurants will help your child avoid becoming overweight. A recent book, *Eat this, not that! for kids!*, offers food choices that help to minimize the damage done in these establishments.

Another word of caution: when shopping for foods, don't be fooled by labels. Many Red foods are promoted as being healthy with terms like "low fat," "all natural," or "no transfats." The idea that a food is healthy may promote overeating. One study found that moviegoers ate 49 percent more granola (84 extra calories) when the package label said "low fat" compared with moviegoers who were given the exact same granola without "low fat" on the label.

Dr. Brian Wansink is a Cornell University professor who has done dozens of ingenious studies exploring the reasons why we eat. He proposed a simple rule for meal planning. He calls it the "Half-Plate Rule," which simply means that, for lunch and dinner, half of the plate should be vegetables and fruit (Green), while the other half is protein and carbs (mostly Yellow). Regardless of the strategy you choose, the goal should be to increase consumption of fruits and vegetables in your child's diet.

## How to Eat

A recent University of Pennsylvania study showed that eating rapidly could contribute to childhood obesity. The researchers videotaped four-year-old children eating a meal with their parents and calculated the number of mouthfuls of food per minute the kids were consuming. When the kids were weighed and measured two years later, the children who were fast eaters at age four were more likely to be overweight at age six. On average, the four-year-olds who ate four mouthfuls per minute were about four times as likely to become overweight as kids who ate two mouthfuls per minute.

I'm a good example of the hazards of eating quickly since I was a fast eater as a kid. My dad was a high school science teacher who also taught at a night school. His evening classes started at 7:00. Dinners were always rushed so he could leave by 6:30. Eating quickly probably helped me become an overweight child. It's been a hard habit to break. As an adult, I've had to make a deliberate effort to catch myself when I'm gobbling my food. It would have been a lot easier to learn to eat slowly when I was a child.

Consider the atmosphere at mealtime in your home. Does it feel rushed or relaxed? If it's rushed, what is everyone in a hurry to do? Can you rearrange schedules so that there's more time to eat? Is there anything else that increases the stress at dinnertime so that you just want to eat quickly to get it over with? Turning off the TV and reducing other distractions (see Step 4) will help to create a more relaxed atmosphere.

Review your child's eating behaviors. You don't need to videotape him and count the number of mouthfuls per minute, but quietly observe how your child eats. When his mouth is full is he preparing the next mouthful so that he can put it in his mouth as soon as he has swallowed? Is he chewing rapidly so that he can swallow and put more food in his mouth?

If your child is inhaling his food, there are several things you can do to help him develop a healthier eating style. First, examine the pace of your eating. If you're rushing, your child will too, so you'll need to slow down. Pause after each mouthful. Put your fork or spoon down between mouthfuls. Towards the middle of the meal, put your utensils down and just converse for a minute before starting to eat again.

If you are eating at a relaxed pace but your kids are still eating too fast, there are several things you can do. For younger children, you can playfully suggest eating with your non-dominant hand. You can say something like, "We always eat with the fork in our right hand. I wonder what would happen if we ate with our left hand?"

Older kids will require a more subtle approach. They might rebel if you just tell them to "slow down," but if you're having a conversation, the pace of eating usually slows down. If your child is reluctant to talk, don't ask so many questions that it turns into an interrogation. Instead you and your spouse could have a conversation about a topic that would interest your child, and after a few minutes, ask him what he thinks.

## Action Plan

1. I will find out which fruits my child likes best and make them available (where)_____ and (when)_____.

2. I will choose a Red food that we frequently eat and reduce the frequency from _____ times per week to _____ times per week. I will substitute _____ for the Red food.

3. I will limit meals at fast food restaurants to no more than _____ times per week.

4. I will limit sodas and other sugary drinks to no more than one can per day and replace them with_____.

5. If my child is a fast eater, I will try to slow the pace of eating by _____ _____.

# Step 4: Create a Healthy Eating Environment

In one study Dr. Brian Wansink found that people made an average of 221 food decisions every day. Most of these eating decisions don't result from physical hunger but, rather, eating is usually triggered by subtle environmental cues. Something as simple as the size of the plate can determine how much food will be consumed. After we've reviewed some of the triggers for eating, you'll be able to make small changes in your household to reduce the number of those triggers so that there will be less unnecessary eating.

Before your child starts school you have almost complete control over her environment. As your child grows up she'll spend more time away from home, but you'll still be able to influence some of her eating decisions.

Perhaps the most obvious cue that triggers eating is the sight of food, or the sight of other people eating. Have you ever seen a commercial on TV for an appetizing food and then found yourself wandering into the kitchen searching for something to eat even though you'd just had dinner? Or perhaps you've had a meal and then visited friends who were eating and made a split-second decision to join them for dessert. From TV commercials, pictures in magazines, seeing a fast-food restaurant as you drive by, to the bowl of candies on a co-worker's desk, we're never far from a visual food cue.

While a TV commercial for a tantalizing treat is an obvious cue, often the trigger that makes us eat isn't immediately apparent. Betsy, a 48-year-old teacher, was in the habit of using the drive-thru window at Taco Bell to get a burrito for a snack while she was on the way home from school. She said she needed the snack to "tide me over until dinner." One day, they were doing road work near her school so she had to take a detour to get home. She didn't drive by the Taco Bell and didn't have the burrito. When she sat down to dinner that night it occurred to her that she hadn't had her afternoon snack and didn't miss it. Betsy hadn't realized that her daily burrito wasn't prompted by physical hunger but rather by a powerful visual cue, the sight of the restaurant.

Like Betsy, the dozens of intelligent, well-educated people in Dr. Wansink's studies ate more in response to an external cue but didn't recognize the effect that cue had on their eating. You and I are susceptible to these hidden triggers whether we recognize them or not. Your child isn't immune to the power of food cues either. To help reduce mindless eating you'll need to reduce the number of these cues at home and help your child become more aware of his eating.

With a little planning you can alter your home to reduce the number of cues he will encounter. Once you recognize the general idea, you can examine your home to reduce these cues. Here are a few suggestions to get you started:

- Keep all the food in the kitchen — remove snacks and treats from the living room and the rest of the house. Don't let your kids keep food in their bedroom.
- If you must have high-calorie treats in the house, keep them out of sight. Put them in opaque containers on high shelves, or in the back of the refrigerator.
- Make eating a singular activity, preferably in one place. Have your child turn off the TV or computer, and come to the table to sit and eat.

51

- If you think your child's request for something to eat was prompted by an external cue, ask her if she's really feeling hungry in her tummy or if she just wants to eat because of something she's seen.
- Serve food from the kitchen rather than putting the food on the table and allowing your child to serve himself. If he wants more, he can go to the kitchen to get more.

Research has shown that the more effort it takes to get food, the less we'll eat. In one classic study, obese people ate more almonds if they were shelled but not if they were still in the shells. In another study secretaries, ate about nine Hershey's Kisses if they were in a bowl on their desks, but only ate four if the bowl was on a file cabinet six feet away. Having to crack open the shells or get up and walk six feet decreased eating. Now think about the high-calorie foods in your house. How can you make them more difficult (but not impossible) to get?

It may seem that the results of changing the food cues in your home would have a trivial effect on your child's weight. It's true that you won't see any noticeable weight loss overnight, but if you are consistent you can expect long-term results. For example, if the secretaries kept the Kisses on the file cabinet instead of their desks, they'd lose more than a pound in six weeks, or almost nine pounds in a year. Small changes over time add up to big differences.

## Eating Mindfully

For the secretaries, getting up to get the Kisses required some effort but also created a brief interlude between the urge to eat and getting the food. The time between urge and opportunity gave them a chance to decide if they really wanted the Kisses. Some of the time they decided that they didn't need to eat. When you can stop and make a deliberate decision about eating instead of eating automatically in response to a cue, you may decide that eating isn't necessary. You can show your child how this is done by being a good role model.

If you have a young child, have you ever noticed how often she copies what you do? If Mom is vacuuming, it's likely that your young daughter will want to vacuum too. Little boys may pretend to shave like their dads. Teens will see their same sex parent as a model even if they are rebellious and make a point of trying to do things differently. What eating behaviors are you modeling for your child? If you eat while working at your desk, driving, reading the paper, watching TV, or talking on the phone, you are modeling distracted eating. You're teaching your kids that eating is a mindless, automatic behavior that doesn't warrant their full attention. With enough repetitions, the activities that have been paired with eating will lead to cravings to eat.

To increase mindfulness, you can help your child by focusing on the sensations that the food provides. Occasionally you could bite into a carrot and comment on the noise it makes, or ask your child if he knows what you're cooking from the smell. You could comment on the spices you used to season a dish and ask your child if it's too spicy or too salty. The immediate goal is to increase your child's awareness of the food he is eating. When eating becomes less automatic and a more conscious, deliberate act you'll have increased the likelihood that, some of the time, your child will decide that he really doesn't want to eat.

## Action Plan

1. I will remove all food from rooms other than the kitchen and dining room.

2. I will serve from the kitchen. If my child wants seconds he can go into the kitchen to get the additional food.

3. We will make eating a singular activity instead of eating while doing other things.

4. I will wrap leftovers in aluminum foil rather than clear plastic wrap, or store them in opaque rather than glass containers.

5. I will make it more difficult to eat high-calorie foods by _____
   _____.

6. I will help my children eat mindfully by _____
   _____
   _____.

# Step 5: Avoid Portion Distortion

The Centers for Disease Control estimates that American children consume 150 more calories each day than kids did in 1989. Research published in the *Journal of the American Dietetic Association* found that larger portions were responsible for most of the increase in the number of calories kids were putting away. Since Americans of all ages eat too much, you will need to monitor the size of your child's portions when eating in restaurants and at home.

## Eating Out, Eating In

Several years ago the movie *Supersize Me* illustrated the disastrous effects of consuming large portions of fast food. For a month, Morgan Spurlock, the documentary filmmaker, ate only at McDonald's and, whenever it was offered, he was obligated to have a supersized portion. He routinely ate 500-calorie servings of French fries accompanied by 42-ounce Cokes. At the end of the month he had gained 25 pounds and was suffering from liver dysfunction and depression. While it's unlikely that you or your kids will try a similar stunt, no one is immune to the effects of increasing portion sizes.

McDonald's and all the other fast food restaurants make it easy to eat more than we need. Usually a significantly larger portion is priced insignificantly more than the smaller size so it's hard to resist a "bargain." The weight your child gains comes cheaply, but considering the medical costs of obesity, supersizing might not be such a good deal.

While sit-down restaurants usually don't offer an option to supersize their dinners, the portions served are still too large. For example, the owner of an upscale New York restaurant noted, "Our average portion of fish is 13 ounces." Ideally, a serving of fish should be three ounces, or about the size of a checkbook. He went on to say, "Restaurants serving minute portions have gone out of business." Not surprisingly, many restaurants have increased the amount of food they serve. In a Penn State study, diners at a cafeteria were served either a standard portion of pasta or a portion that was one-and-a-half times as large. Having a large portion resulted in an extra 172 calories, even though many of the diners weren't aware that they had eaten more food.

If you order a typical meal at a nice restaurant, you'll eat too much even if you go easy on the bread. The best solution, one that I've frequently used, is to order one dinner and an extra salad and split it. If you've got two or more kids, it may take some negotiating to find a meal that they both like and can split. If this is impossible, you can ask for a "doggie bag" when the food is served and put the excess in the bag BEFORE starting to eat.

While it's easy to see the role that restaurants play in increasing our eating, the same trend is at work at home. In the last few years we've come to expect larger portions wherever we eat. For example, a typical bagel 20 years ago was three inches in diameter and had 140 calories. Now the bagel that you put in your toaster is about six inches across and has 350 calories. One study looked at the size of portions of homemade foods. In a 20-year interval, homemade cheeseburgers grew from 333 calories to 590 calories, Mexican food servings added 133 calories, and desserts grew by 55 calories. Another study compared the caloric content of recipes in the first edition of *Joy of Cooking* published in 1936 with recipes in the 2006 edition of this classic cookbook. In 1936 servings averaged 268 calories, while in 2006 they averaged 436 calories per serving. Whether we're eating at an all-you-can eat buffet, a fast food outlet, or in our own dining room, the portions are too large.

While girls are supposed to eat sparingly, parents often take pride in their son's ability to consume large portions of food. I recall one of my father's friends describing his family's visit to an all-you-can eat buffet. With pride he recounted how his 11-year-old son made so many trips back to the buffet table that the server asked, "Are you going to eat all that?" Small portions are lady-like; boys are manlier if they eat huge quantities of food.

## Resigning From the "Clean Plate Club"

We've grown accustomed to eating more than we need. You can help reverse this trend in your family. Let your kids see you serving yourself reasonable portions and occasionally leaving a little food on the plate because you're full so you've stopped eating. Don't worry about "wasting" food; the extra fat on your waist would be more wasteful. If you're worried about the starving children in a third-world country write a check to a charity rather than eating more food.

If you serve smaller portions, will your kids go hungry? It's unlikely. Recognize that no one in your family is in danger of starvation. It's been estimated that an adult of normal weight could go for several months without eating and survive, so you're not endangering anyone's health by reducing portion size. Also, don't estimate correct portion size based on the amount of food your child will eat. One study found that, on average, we eat 92 percent of the food that is given to us, so just because your child will eat three hamburgers doesn't mean he needs or even wants three hamburgers; but many kids will eat them just because they're there.

Don't be afraid that your children will complain if you reduce the amount you serve. In one of Dr. Wansink's studies, a 20 percent reduction of the size of the portion went unnoticed. If you think that your child might object or complain about being hungry, proceed gradually; don't make drastic reductions in portion size overnight. If your child complains after finishing the smaller portion, have him wait for a few minutes then ask if he's still hungry. Most likely, he'll have forgotten about more food but if he still says he's hungry, he can get up, go into the kitchen and serve himself.

If you've followed through with your Step 2 Action Plan you should be having more sit-down dinners as a family. Still, with our hectic lifestyles, there may be some dinners where your kids serve themselves, often by just grabbing whatever they can find in the refrigerator. With this kind of unstructured eating, a child may have difficulty accurately judging portion size. A possible solution is for you to prepare a plate for your child so all she has to do is take it from the refrigerator, remove the cellophane wrap, and put it in the microwave. Although not ideal, you'll provide some structure to the meal and help control portion size.

## Eating With Your Eyes

One simple change you can make to help your child be comfortable with smaller servings is to use smaller plates and glasses. Several studies have demonstrated that adults and kids eat more when they use big plates. In one of these studies adults were given either medium-sized bowls (17 ounce) or large bowls (34 ounce) and allowed to take as much ice cream as they wanted. Not surprisingly, the folks with the big bowls took 31 percent more and consumed an average of 127 extra calories. Plate size also affects judgment. If you serve a piece of pie on a large plate, people will underestimate the number of calories it has when compared to the same piece of pie served on a small plate.

An easy way to eat less without feeling deprived is to use smaller plates. Right now, before you forget, go into your kitchen and measure the diameter of your everyday dinner plates. You'll probably find that they're about 12 inches across. Perhaps it's time to donate them to Goodwill and buy a smaller set. If this seems impractical, you could always use your salad plates for the main meal. While you're re-equipping your kitchen, take a look at the glasses you use. Drinking from wide glasses usually results in more consumption than drinking from tall thin glasses, so you may need to replace them too.

Here are some guidelines from the National Institute of Health to help you judge reasonable portion sizes:

Cereal: clenched fist (1 cup)
Pancake: compact disc
Cheese: 2 slices (1 ½ oz.)
Baked potato: clenched fist
Cooked rice or pasta: ½ baseball (1/2 cup)
Meat or poultry: deck of cards (3 oz.)
Peanut butter: ping-pong ball (2 tbsp.)
Ice Cream: ½ baseball (1/2 cup)

## Red Food Portion Control

You shouldn't feel guilty when you reduce the portion size of high-calorie treats since most of the enjoyment comes with the first few bites. The easiest way of cutting back on treats is to buy them in single-serving packages. For example, rather than keeping a half-gallon of ice cream in the freezer, buy ice cream sandwiches, cones, pops, or cups. When you're eating ice cream from a half-gallon tub, portion size isn't defined so it's easy to eat more. When you're having an ice cream sandwich you know that, when the sandwich is finished, you've had your portion. Likewise, if you are going to buy cookies, chips or other treats, try to buy them in single-serving packages. It may be cheaper to buy cookies by the bag instead of in snack packs, but getting cheaper calories might be a bargain you can live without. If snack packs aren't available, you can buy the larger package and use baggies to make single servings. You can reduce the temptation to sneak extra servings by labeling each pack. Write the child's name on the packs that he is entitled to for the coming week.

A word of caution: for prepared foods, the portion size listed on the label can be misleading. For example, one snack package of chocolate chip cookies listed 200 calories per portion. You'd have to read the label carefully to determine that a portion was just one of the two cookies in the package. It would be easy to eat both assuming that you've consumed 200 rather than 400 calories.

### Action Plan

1. When we go out to eat, I will avoid restaurants that serve buffet-style.

2. At fast food restaurants, I'll go online to get nutrition information to encourage healthier choices. I won't order super-sized portions unless I will share them with two or more people.

3. At sit-down restaurants, I'll have my children split meals or ask for a doggie bag when ordering so I can take the excess food home.

4. I will serve meals using smaller plates and glasses.

5. If my child says he's still hungry, I'll have him wait a few minutes then ask, "Are you still hungry," before offering more food.

6. For treats and snack foods, I'll buy single-serving packages.

# Step 6: Don't Use Food as a Reward or to Soothe Unpleasant Feelings

Kristen, a 48-year-old dietitian, was a participant at a continuing education workshop I was leading. She offered an example of how food was used to soothe unpleasant feelings. A few weeks earlier, she was spending the night at her friend Barbara's house. Barbara, a middle-aged woman weighing 195 pounds, was eating Ben and Jerry's ice cream from the container while they were watching TV. The phone rang. It was Kristen's adult daughter calling to tell Kristen that the daughter's husband was filing for divorce. Barbara saw that Kristen was upset so without hesitation, she said, "Here," and offered Kristen the container and spoon. As a child Barbara had learned that eating a favorite food makes you feel better when you are upset so she was offering the ice cream to comfort her friend. Unfortunately, it's very easy to teach your child the same lesson.

Most of us have a long history of having food associated with love. As infants, regardless of whether we were breast or bottle-fed, we were held and comforted while eating. Typically, this was a warm, loving time with our mother (or father) paying attention to us and frequently smiling, singing, cooing, or just rocking us while we were eating. Being held while nursing (or drinking formula from a bottle) is one of the most important bonding experiences for an infant, but as the child develops there should be fewer connections between eating and nurturing.

When an infant cries, parents often assume that she is hungry and offer food when she may not be hungry at all. She might be crying because she is frightened, cold, or just needs her diaper changed, but this pairing of feeding with being comforted may be the beginning of a lifelong pattern of using food to feel better whenever there's any emotional distress.

Learning to associate eating with emotions continues throughout childhood and adolescence. Consider Alyssa N. When she was two, her mother divorced her father because he had bipolar (manic-depressive) disorder, couldn't hold a job, and occasionally had hallucinations and angry outbursts. Alyssa lived with her mother but, when Mrs. N. remarried and had another child, Alyssa felt abandoned. Alyssa sensed that she was an afterthought; all of her mother's attention was focused on her new husband and baby. Alyssa's father was no help. When he did call, he was needy, asking for Alyssa's support in his continuing conflict with his ex-wife. Throughout her childhood the one source of love and understanding was Alyssa's Greek grandmother.

Whenever she could, Alyssa went straight from school to her grandmother's house. Grandma comforted and nurtured Alyssa and gave her all the treats she wasn't allowed to have at home. She was praised, held, kissed and offered ice cream, cupcakes, and, of course, baklava at Grandma's. Alyssa spent the whole summer between second and third grade at her grandmother's house and gained 20 pounds. After her grandmother died, Alyssa was depressed and occasionally would eat so much she became sick. Fast forward 30 years: Alyssa now weighs 260 pounds and, when she is alone on evenings and weekends, binges on many of the same sugary treats her grandmother once provided.

## Preventing Emotional Eating

When you were a kid, did your parents offer you ice cream or some other treat when you fell off your bicycle and were crying? On a rainy Saturday afternoon, if you were bored and restless, did your dad offer to take you out for pizza or ice cream? Maybe it seemed that the only time you got your busy mom's undivided attention was when the two of you were cooking together.

Now that you are a parent, have you ever:

- offered your child a treat to cheer her up after a disappointment?
- taken your child out for a special treat to reward an accomplishment at school or elsewhere?
- promised your child a special treat after enduring an unpleasant experience, like going to the dentist or getting an injection?

Being a good parent requires that you nurture your child when he's upset, but there is no reason to assume that nurturance requires food. You can console or soothe your child without using food. Give some thought to other treats that don't involve eating, which you can use to reward or soothe your child. Instead of a trip to the ice cream parlor, how about offering your child the chance to do something special with Mom or Dad, or a privilege that's usually reserved for older children? For a younger child, it can be as simple as sitting and reading to your child, or letting him stay up later on a weekend to watch a TV program. An older child might like a song downloaded from iTunes more than an ice cream cone. Sometimes, just acknowledging the feeling that your child is experiencing along with a hug is enough.

### Recognizing Emotional Eating

Many parents are familiar with the link between emotional upsets and eating for themselves, but it may be more difficult to see when kids do the same thing. For example, emotional eating was demonstrated in a recent English study of 4,000 teens. Over a five-year period the teens reporting more stress had higher BMIs and larger waistlines.

Eating, usually a high-calorie treat, is often used to soothe unpleasant emotions like sadness, anxiety, anger, boredom, and loneliness but sometimes eating can be used to increase the good feelings when we're happy. Getting to the root cause of negative feelings isn't always easy. Children may not be able to verbalize how they're feeling and often they can't change their environment to reduce their emotional distress, so eating is an easy, convenient way to feel better. If she feels bad, comfort can be found in the kitchen!

If your child has already developed a pattern of using food to cope with emotions, the first step is to recognize the emotions she is experiencing. You can then help her to deal with the emotion directly rather than trying to avoid it by eating. The **Emotions That May Trigger Eating** chart will help you identify what your child is feeling so that you'll be able to suggest alternatives to eating.

## Emotions That May Trigger Eating

| Emotion | Definition | Physical clues | Mental clues |
|---|---|---|---|
| **Depression,** also: sad, down, blue, bummed | Unhappy feelings following loss: often loss of self-esteem after being teased | Tears, whining, slower movement, tiredness, increased body pain | Thoughts of guilt, worthlessness, shame, hopelessness |
| **Anxiety,** also: stress, afraid, tense, worried | Unrealistic fears, uneasiness, apprehensive-ness about something that will happen in the future | Increased heart rate, sweating, difficulty breathing, "butterflies" in the stomach | Thinking something awful is going to happen, may be specific ("the plane will crash") or just vague uneasiness |
| **Anger,** also: mad, hostile, annoyed, irritated, pissed-off | Strong feelings that you have been injured, treated unfairly, or threatened | Stiffening of the body, clenched jaw, increased blood pressure | Striking out or attacking, thinking of getting revenge, thinking about the incident repeatedly |
| **Boredom,** also: monotonous, dullness | Distress resulting from a lack of stimulation or repetition of uninteresting activities | Restlessness, fidgeting, yawning | Thinking time seems to pass slowly, frequent daydreaming, being easily distracted |
| **Loneliness** also: isolation, aloneness | Distress resulting from lack of satisfying social relationships | Avoidance of social situations, awkwardness around others | Thinking that you have been abandoned or rejected by others |
| **Happiness** also: joy, cheerful, elated, upbeat, euphoric | Highly pleasant state of well-being and contentment | Smiling, laughing, extra energy or drive, outgoing | Positive, optimistic thoughts, increased self-esteem |

Some emotional eating patterns are quite common among overweight kids. Being teased, for example, often elicits depression and loneliness that is then soothed with food. Latchkey kids often spend several hours after school each day by themselves and may use food to cope with boredom and loneliness. Teen-age girls may become anxious anticipating a dance or other social activity and then go on a restrictive diet that is followed by binge eating.

If you've identified an emotional eating pattern, help your child understand why she is eating. Depending on her age, you could ask, "Are you really hungry, or are you feeling sad?" or "Sometimes when Mommy (or Daddy) is feeling, nervous I feel like I want to eat something. Is that how you're feeling now?" When you've identified the emotional eating pattern, the two of you can find an alternative to eating. For example, you could ask, "When you're feeling sad, would it help to listen to your favorite music?"

Although emotional eating is most often associated with negative feelings like sadness and stress, sometimes eating follows happy feelings. Most celebrations involve food. It's hard to visualize a birthday party without cake or a family Thanksgiving without turkey and stuffing. Since eating is an essential part of these good times, it's not surprising that when we want to feel good, or make someone else feel good, we use food. I'm certainly not suggesting that we remove all of the pleasant experiences associated with eating. In our efforts to encourage healthy eating, we shouldn't deprive our kids of common fun experiences with food. If the soccer team is going out to celebrate, it would stigmatize your child to prevent her from going. If the celebratory eating is in a social setting, it might be useful to suggest limits in portion size

*It's NOT Just Baby Fat!*

beforehand, but otherwise encourage your child to participate.

## Action Plan

1. When my child is crying or visibly upset, I won't offer food, but will soothe him by _____
_____.

2. When I want to reward my child or celebrate her accomplishments, I will suggest _____ instead of eating.

3. If my child is home alone after school, I will _____ _____ to minimize his loneliness.

4. If I identify an emotional eating pattern, I will _____.

# Step 7: Make Sure Your Child is Getting Enough Sleep

If you're like many adults, you don't consider sleeping habits when thinking about your child's weight or your own. Unfortunately, about half of American adults don't get the recommended seven to nine hours, and many are proud of their ability to function on little sleep. If you're among the sleep deprived, consider what happens to you when you're tired. Most likely you don't have energy and you don't feel well. So, what do you do to make yourself feel better and increase your energy? Many people reach for something to eat, especially something that is rich in sugar to get a boost of energy. If this is your pattern, it's important for you and for your kids to change your thinking about sleep. Recognize that sleep is NOT a luxury that ambitious people can't afford. Sleep is a biological necessity and lack of sleep is unhealthy and can cause weight gain. One study of adult women suggested that chronic sleeplessness could be responsible for between six to twelve extra pounds.

With all the emphasis on eating and exercise, few parents recognize that sleeping can also affect their child's weight. A recent review of 11 studies of sleep and weight in children found unanimous agreement that short sleep duration was associated with increased likelihood of obesity. The results were similar regardless if the studies had been conducted in the U.S., Japan, Brazil, or France, although several studies reported a greater link between obesity and sleep loss for boys than for girls. One study found the odds of obesity increased five-fold for each hour of missed sleep!

Although the link between childhood obesity and sleep deprivation has been convincingly demonstrated, the cause isn't clear. Animal studies show that lack of sleep results in increased eating. For humans, the increased eating is primarily of foods high in fat and carbohydrates. There may be a physiological reason for this. Sleep deprivation lowers levels of leptin and increases ghrelin. Leptin is a hormone secreted by fat that acts as an appetite suppressor while ghrelin is a hormone produced in the stomach when it is empty signaling hunger. If you don't sleep enough, you get two physiological signals that you need more to eat.

Unfortunately, about half of American school kids don't get enough sleep. Here are the recommended sleep guidelines for kids:

Newborns (1–2 months): 10 ½–18 hours
Infants (3-11 months): 9-12 hours at night and 1–4 naps during the day
Toddlers (1–3 years): 12–14 hours including one daytime nap
Preschoolers (3–5 years): 11–13 hours
School-aged (5–12 years): 10–11 hours
Teens: 8-9 hours

What can you do to help your child get enough sleep?

- For most kids, it's helpful to establish a regular sleep schedule for weeknights, allowing somewhat later bedtimes on weekends.
- Avoid going to bed hungry or too full. A light snack before bedtime is okay.
- Discourage using the bed for anything other than sleeping.
- Don't let your child sleep with pets.

- If your child wakes up in the middle of the night, try to avoid bright lights, which can make it more difficult to get back to sleep.
- Colas and other caffeinated drinks should be avoided in the afternoon and evening.
- Schedule any exercise or workout sessions no later than three hours before bedtime.

For all children, the bedroom should be conducive to sleep with no distractions. Watching TV right before bedtime may increase resistance to going to sleep. Temptations like video games and televisions should be removed from the child's bedroom (more about this later).

Toddlers may feel more secure if they take a favorite stuffed animal or blanket to bed with them. For preschool children, a quiet bedtime routine helps prepare the child for sleep. Reading a bedtime story is a tried-and-true method that gives the child a feeling of security before going to sleep while offering the parent an opportunity to be with the child without distractions.

For teens, getting enough sleep is especially difficult. You may have tried to get your teen to go to bed earlier and met with resistance. Several parents have told me that, no matter how much they've reminded, nagged, or bribed, their kids just wouldn't go to bed any earlier. These parents didn't realize that they were fighting their kids' biological clocks.

With puberty teenagers' internal clocks get set back so that the "natural" time to go to sleep is later, usually around 11 p.m. This means that teens won't get enough sleep, especially if they have to be in school by 8:00 the next morning. Setting a 10 p.m. bedtime on school nights is a reasonable compromise. With accumulating sleep deficits, your son or daughter may want to sleep late on the weekends to catch up, but sleeping more than an extra hour or two may disrupt your child's sleep cycle, making it harder for him or her to go to bed on weeknights.

While you can't control when your teen's school day starts, you can encourage quiet time in the evening, limiting loud music, the use of computers, phones and instant messaging close to bedtime.

### Action Plan

1. For younger children, I will establish a bedtime routine. At _____ o'clock, we will stop other activities and, instead _____ for _____minutes before turning off the lights.

2. For older kids, TV, computer games, etc. will be off by ___ o'clock on school nights. If my child resists sleeping, I will encourage _____ until he is sleepy.

3. For teens, I will discuss evening rituals with my daughter to help her arrange her schedule so that she can be in bed by 10 on weeknights.

# Step 8: Encourage Physical Activity

Marshall was a slender, exceptionally fit 35-year-old professor at a prestigious West Coast university. He was an avid bicyclist, and enjoyed riding 50 miles several times a week with his pals. At 5 feet, 11, he weighed 167 pounds, but several years earlier he was almost 100 pounds heavier. I asked Marshall how he managed such a significant weight loss. Tracing his weight history revealed the importance of early parental support for physical activity.

When Marshall was in junior high, his mother started a new job that required a long commute. She wasn't home for dinner and his dad didn't like to cook so they relied on fast food and take-out for many of their meals. Marshall gained weight. When he was in college, he lived in the dorm and took his meals at the all-you-can-eat cafeteria. He gained more weight. In grad school, he became concerned about the health risks of his excess weight as well as the not-so-subtle rejection he was getting from the ladies. Fortunately, a friend who was into biking, persuaded Marshall to join him. Marshall was hooked, and bicycling became an almost daily routine.

I was especially curious as to how Marshall went from being a sedentary teen and college student to an active adult. Although he credited his grad school friend for providing the impetus to ride bikes, Marshall recognized that it was his father who set the stage for his love of bicycling. When he was a child his father would take Marshall and his brother on long bike rides around their city. Marshall never saw this activity as "exercise" or something he had to do to lose weight; it was just having a good time with Dad. Twenty years later, when his friend invited him to ride, it again was just for fun.

## Examine Your Exercise Attitude

Most kids don't have parents who are willing to ride bikes with them. This is unfortunate since one study showed that kids who had active parents were six times as likely to become active themselves. Although sedentary parents might encourage their child to "get some exercise," they rarely get active with their kids. Often a parent who is inactive feels guilty about her sedentary lifestyle, so focusing on her child's lack of activity seems hypocritical. It's just easier to avoid the whole subject and rely on the child's gym class to provide the exercise he needs. Unfortunately, 90 percent of elementary schools don't provide daily P.E. classes, and only about a third of high school kids get daily gym class. In California, the state law mandates 20 minutes a day of physical activity, but less than half of the schools comply with this requirement.

You may have mixed feelings about exercise. You may feel that you don't have time to exercise, or that it's boring, or even that you hate to sweat. If your past experiences in gym classes or team sports were unpleasant, you want to protect your children from similar experiences, but don't let your bad experiences carry over to your children. Like Marshall's dad, you can go for bike rides with your son, or play ball with your daughter, dance with your son, go for a hike in the woods, swim in a pool, or just walk around the block. The important thing is that your child sees you being active and is being active himself. If the two of you are enjoying yourselves, the good feelings of spending time with a parent will become associated with physical activity.

At a workshop I was leading, Maria, a 42-year-old mother of two, told me about her experiences in her middle school gym class. Coming from a traditional

Hispanic family, she was modest, so changing in the girls' locker room was uncomfortable for her. Her uneasiness grew to active avoidance after several girls started teasing her about her "bubble butt" when she was wearing gym shorts. She pleaded with her mother to write a note excusing her from gym class for the rest of the semester. Her uneasiness with exercise has continued throughout her adulthood. Now that she is a mother, she doesn't object when Theresa, her nine-year-old daughter, watches TV rather than going out to play.

Examine your past experiences with exercise. Were you:

- embarrassed because you had to wear revealing clothing like a swimsuit, gym shorts, or a leotard?
- stressed because everyone was watching you when playing a sport (for example, being at bat in a baseball game, or making a foul shot in basketball)?
- humiliated when you were the last one chosen for a team?
- embarrassed when you couldn't keep up with your group on a hike or perform an activity everyone else was doing?
- feeling awkward, clumsy or uncoordinated when playing a sport?

If you've had any of these experiences, it's quite likely that you now avoid exercising, and you may be communicating your dislike to your child.

Perhaps you've tried to lose weight by exercising and found that it didn't work, so why put your child through the same disappointment? Did you join a gym and drop out or try running but found it too difficult? The unfortunate reality is that it's very difficult to lose weight by exercise alone and, for most people, the amount of time and effort required makes it unrealistic to try. Nonetheless, there is evidence that, over time, increased physical activity can result in weight loss, and exercise is necessary to maintain weight loss. So, even if you could lose weight by dieting alone, you'd need to become active to maintain the loss. Still, if you are discouraged with your own efforts to lose weight by exercising, recognize that by helping your child become more active you will minimize her future weight gain.

Regardless of your own experiences, it's important to help your child develop good exercise habits. One simple change parents can make is to praise their child for being active, regardless of the child's athletic abilities. A study of middle-school kids in Pennsylvania confirmed that the children who had been criticized by their families or their peers for their lack of abilities were less likely to play sports or be physically active. Since most children are acutely sensitive to their parents' reactions, it's important not to let your disappointment show if your child lacks athletic skill. This can be a challenge, especially if there is another child in the family who has athletic abilities. It will take a deliberate effort to avoid making comparisons between the children.

Praising poor performance will seem inauthentic, even to the youngest child, but realistic praise for effort can help motivate your child. Simple phrases like "you're getting better," or "I like it when you really make an effort," will be rewarding even if she isn't a star athlete.

On the other hand, parents who were good athletes may have different problems if their kids don't share their enthusiasm. You'd like your daughter to share the enjoyment you had when you played your sport, but she is reluctant to get involved. It's disappointing if your child is sedentary and doesn't enjoy sports when you found it so rewarding. Mark, a 42-year-old father of two was a "jock" in high school. He was pleased with his youngest son's enthusiasm for baseball and football, but he was worried about Jason, his older son.

Jason was a sixth grader who was a good student and was thoroughly involved with his hobby, performing magic tricks. Learning a new trick was time consuming. He spent hours in his room practicing over and over until he could do the sleight of hand without being detected. When he wasn't practicing, often he was on the computer watching other magicians on YouTube videos. Jason's parents were concerned because he was gaining weight, and because magic was a solitary activity, he was becoming isolated. Mark tried to get Jason involved in sports. When the other kids were outside tossing the football, Mark told Jason he should go out and join the game. When Jason resisted, Mark threatened to curtail Jason's computer or TV time. A few times Mark offered to pay Jason a dollar if he'd play ball with the other kids. None of these interventions worked. Jason still refused, or if he were forced to go outside, he'd just stand on the sidelines and watch the other kids play.

If your child is like Jason and prefers video games, computers, television, reading or other sedentary activities to sports, there may be a reason for his reluctance. Since sports involve other kids, there might be conflict or other hassles between kids that your child would rather avoid so he doesn't participate. Or your child could have performance anxiety. Perhaps he's afraid that he'll strike out, drop the ball, or embarrass himself because he lacks the physical strength or coordination to perform well. Rather than risk humiliation, he chooses not to play. Your child might be more willing to participate in an individual sport because, without teammates, there are fewer social pressures. Swimming, track, karate, gymnastics or skiing could be good choices.

If your child adamantly refuses to participate in sports, would he join a group like Boy Scouts? Boy or Girl Scouts frequently have outdoor activities like hiking, camping, and canoeing that don't require any particular physical skill but do provide exercise. If your child is reluctant to get involved, why not plan family outings that include these outdoor activities, and ask your child to invite a friend.

## NEAT is Neat; Sitting Isn't

NEAT is the acronym for Non-Exercise Activity Thermogenisis, which is just a fancy way of describing the movement of your body when you're not exercising. Your body needs energy (calories) to maintain itself. Breathing, circulating blood, digesting, and other bodily functions use energy. The energy required to maintain your body is your basal metabolism. You also need energy for vigorous exercise like running or playing sports. NEAT refers to everything in-between basal metabolism and exercise. Standing, walking, clapping your hands at a concert, fidgeting, and crossing your legs while sitting are all examples of non-exercise activity thermogenisis. Even gum chewing uses 12 calories per hour.

If an overweight adult tries to lose weight by increasing NEAT, it's likely that the progress will be so slow that he'll get discouraged and give up. On the other hand, increasing a child's NEAT will help him avoid gaining weight. While fidgeting or riding a bike to school by itself is not likely to compensate for an extra dessert, when you add up all the calories used by NEAT each day, and then look at the results over several years, it would make a substantial difference. Being more active in childhood can help prevent the struggle that adults go through when they try to lose weight later in life. It's unfortunate that most kids get less NEAT today than their parents did. Now is the time to get your child moving!

## The Chair is Not Your Friend

For both adults and children, sitting for long periods of time is unhealthy. Even if your child is active at other times, too much sitting causes problems. Sitting uses fewer calories than standing, chewing gum or fidgeting. Also, when your child's muscles are active various substances, including lipoprotein lipase, are produced that can affect how the body uses sugars and fats. Sitting results in low levels of lipoprotein lipase. This contributes to a slower metabolism and most likely to various health problems, including heart disease.

Examine your child's daily routine to see how you can help to increase her movement. Could she walk the dog, rake leaves, or help wash the car? If your child is addicted to video games, could he play while standing? If she is going to be at the computer for hours, could you require several minutes of activity in-between tasks? When discussing these changes with your child, it's important to adopt the proper mindset. You're not putting your child on a diet or trying to turn her into a competitive athlete, so when you present these suggestions to your child, don't mention "exercise" or discuss them in terms of weight loss. Instead, you are helping your child develop a healthy body.

In addition to decreasing sitting and increasing walking, consider ways for adding movement to your child's daily routine. See if your child has developed any labor-saving rituals and encourage the more active alternative. For example, if your child's bedroom is on the second floor, does she leave things on the stairs to take up later? You could make a rule that nothing can be left on the stairs.

## Adding Steps

One study of six- to twelve-year-old children found that girls need 12,000 steps each day, while boys need 15,000 steps to stay at a healthy weight. Thirty years ago 80 percent of kids walked to school. Now only ten percent do. Look at your child's routine to see how you can increase the number of steps. Start by examining how often you drive to take your child someplace. How many of these outings could be accomplished on foot or by riding a bike? If you took turns with another parent, could you walk both kids to school rather than driving them?

Several communities in New Zealand started a "walking school bus." The parents take turns being the "driver," walking with their child to the other children's homes and then walking with all the children to school. Not only do the kids (and parents) get some exercise, but also Mom and Dad avoid the annoying traffic jams that develop around schools. In Marin County, California, a program that included a Walking School Bus, Bike Trains (same idea for bike riding), with frequent-rider contests, and classroom education resulted in a 64 percent increase in the number of children walking and a 114 percent increase in the number of students biking.

One simple way of increasing steps is to use a pedometer. Since Amanda, a 42-year-old mother of two boys, was concerned about her family's weight, she went to a sporting goods store and bought four inexpensive pedometers for herself, her husband Max, and the boys. She kept a chart posted in the kitchen and right before bedtime, everyone recorded the number of steps they had taken that day. At the end of the first week she calculated the average number of daily steps and set a goal of a ten percent increase for the following week. On some weekends she and the boys would plan their walk using a Google map website for walks (http://www.gmap-pedometer.com). The kids enjoyed seeing the satellite view of their route while Amanda and Max checked out the website's calorie calculator for their walk.

When the boys met their weekly goal there was a small reward, usually a privilege like getting to choose which movie they'd rent or staying up later on a weekend night. For Amanda and Max, just meeting their goal and knowing that they were increasing their fitness was reward enough. The ultimate goal was an average of 15,000 steps per day for the boys and 10,000 steps for Amanda and Max.

## Action Plan

1. At least ____ times each week I will offer to _____ (play ball, ride bikes, walk, etc.) with my child.

2. At least ____ times each week, I will be more physically active myself by _____.

3. I will praise my child when he _____ _____.

4. I will examine my child's routine and find _____ activities that she can do by walking or riding a bike.

5. I will buy inexpensive pedometers for the family and post a chart of daily step counts in a prominent place. I will encourage everyone to record their steps daily, and after computing a weekly average,

will offer rewards to the children for each ten percent increase in weekly steps.

# Step 9: Tame Television, Curb Computer Games

The Kaiser Family Foundation reports that kids between eight and eighteen years old average more than seven hours a day, seven days a week, in front of screens. The time spent watching is likely to increase as more kids will have cell phones with media capabilities. For many children, watching TV, playing video games, and using the computer will take up more time than any other activity except, possibly, sleeping. If your family is typical, your kids spend more time in front of screens than you do at a full-time job. It wasn't so long ago that kids spent their spare time playing sports, riding their bikes, or just hanging out with their friends, but now many of these activities have been replaced with time spent staring at screens. How much time does your child spend in front of a monitor or television?

## The Fattening Babysitter

Ten-year-old Brandon was gaining weight, at least in part because of TV. The television was always on in the household. Mrs. S., a stay-at-home mom, kept the TV on to avoid feeling lonely during the day. On weekends, Mr. S. spent his spare time watching (but not playing) sports. A good deal of Brandon's free time was spent in front of the always-on television and meals were always accompanied by the sights and sounds of the tube. If Brandon didn't like what his parents were watching, he could retreat to his bedroom and watch a program on his own TV.

Countless studies have demonstrated the relationship between television viewing and obesity. One national survey suggested that kids who watched a lot of TV were 40 to 50 percent more likely to be overweight. Another study concluded that about 60 percent of all excess weight in children was a result of watching TV. Television and other viewing pastimes contribute to gaining weight several ways. In addition to taking the place of more vigorous free-time activities, there's evidence that your child will use fewer calories watching TV than he would use if he was sitting and reading or even sitting and staring at the wall. Apparently, television viewing DECREASES basal metabolism.

A second way TV adds pounds is that many kids eat while they watch. Dr. Leonard Epstein, a University of Buffalo professor of pediatrics and a leading researcher on childhood obesity, estimates that the average child eats 600 unnecessary calories a day while watching the tube. In addition to snacking while viewing, in many families like Brandon's, the TV is on during mealtimes. A recent study by the Kaiser Family Foundation found that 64 percent of young people said that the television was on during their mealtimes.

Watching TV is a distraction that's likely to result in unnecessary eating. When your child is preoccupied with the program, she's likely to eat more because she's not paying attention to how much she's been consuming. With the TV, on she won't focus on the sensations from her stomach that would tell her she's full and should stop eating. If this becomes a habit, she may lose the ability to accurately judge when she's physically hungry. In addition to eating too much, when the TV is on she won't be thinking about making the healthy food choices that you've been trying to encourage.

What your child is watching also contributes to your child's gaining weight. Children see an average of 40,000 commercials each year; about 7,600 of them will be for candy, fast food, soda, snack foods, and sugary cereals. Very few of the commercials will be for vegetables or other Green foods. A study from the Harvard School of Public Health showed how watching TV can affect children's food choices. The kids who watched more TV ate fewer fruits and vegetables.

So, in addition to being a sedentary activity, television viewing takes the place of more active free-time play, while offering your child the opportunity for unnecessary eating, and encouraging him to make unhealthy food choices. Although busy parents frequently value TV as an inexpensive babysitter for their kids, wouldn't you fire a babysitter that prevented your children from exercising while promoting needless snacking and poor food choices?

If you want to start taming TV, consider where televisions are located in your house. Are there any in your child's bedroom? The Kaiser Family Foundation study found that more than two-thirds of the kids studied had TVs in their bedrooms. Having a television in the child's bedroom promotes weight gain. One study found that kids with TVs in their rooms increased viewing time by 38 minutes per day. Another study of New York kids found that the 40 percent who had a TV in their room were significantly heavier than similar kids who had to watch in the living room or other public areas.

Brandon's parents consulted me because they were concerned about his weight. I approached the topic of television cautiously, starting with the TV set in Brandon's room. When I asked, neither parent could find a reason why Brandon needed his own TV so, with some hesitation, they agreed to move his TV to the basement. Convincing them to turn off the television during meal times was more difficult since it "felt weird" to have silence during meals. It took some time to get used to the occasional quiet during pauses in the conversation, but eventually they found they enjoyed their dinner time discussions without the continual TV background noise. As a fringe benefit, they found that Brandon and his younger brother were calmer during mealtimes. Although Mr. and Mrs. S. weren't willing to turn the TV off at other times, they were pleased that taming TV, along with several of the other steps described in this book, helped Brandon to slim down.

## Beyond Television

In recent years there's been a proliferation of screens in your child's life. In addition to the TV there might be computers, video game consoles, DVD players, smart phones capable of browsing the Internet and, most recently, tablet computers. For many children and adolescents, sports and play have been replaced with more passive activities involving screens.

Larry, an overweight high school sophomore, was referred to me because he was depressed. His parents were worried because he wasn't doing well in school, had few friends and spent most of his free time in his room by himself. Although he wasn't a big TV viewer, he spent every spare minute on the computer playing online video games with teens he'd never met. When he came home from school, Larry would grab a bag of chips and head into his room and only emerge for dinner. At dinner his parents would question him about his homework, so after dinner, Larry would return to his room to do his homework, but most of the evening was spent playing games.

While your child might not be as hooked on video games as Larry was, a recent study conducted in Switzerland showed that playing video games increased the risk of becoming overweight. The researchers found that kids who played video games two or more hours per day were three times as likely to be obese.

Viewing a DVD probably has the same effect as watching TV, but using a computer or playing a video game requires concentration and some movement, if only manipulating the hand-held controller. Often kids move around in their seats while playing. Also, unlike TV viewing, it's difficult to eat while playing a game, and most games have fewer food images and commercials than the typical kids' TV program. Nonetheless, for most video games your child will be sitting, rather than moving and more likely to gain weight.

## What's a Parent to Do?

The Kaiser study found that most parents don't put any limits on the amount of time their children can spend watching TV, using the computer, or playing video games. On the other hand, I've met a few parents who feel so strongly about the negative effects of television that they don't have a TV set in their house. I don't think this is very realistic since kids will watch TV or play games at their friends' houses. Rather than throwing out your TV set or locking the computer, you can set reasonable limits.

The American Academy of Pediatrics recommends that parents limit screen time to two hours per day. They found that parents *can* successfully restrict their children's TV viewing. When the children studied felt that their parents had rules about viewing, they were less likely to exceed the limits and more likely to be physically active. The Kaiser study suggests that it will be easier to set limits for younger kids since there's a big jump in media use for 11- to 14-year-olds, but regardless of your children's age, it will be necessary for you to set firm limits and communicate them clearly to your kids.

What will happen if your children object or just complain, "I'm bored?" Some children seem to have lost the ability to entertain themselves, instead relying on the television, computer, or a video game to fill their free time. As a result, when you start to restrict screen time, they will be uncomfortable, complain, and resist your efforts. As a good parent, you are not required to provide entertainment for every hour your child is awake. Sometimes a little boredom provokes creativity, so if you persist, your child will find something to do, perhaps a physical activity. It may help to remember that there was no television before the 1950s and kids were able to find things to do.

For younger children, one possible compromise is to allow some viewing after a period of active play. A Canadian study found that preteens wearing accelerometers (a device that measures movement) became more active when TV viewing was dependent on reaching a set activity level. After eight weeks these kids were more active, had lower fat intake, ate fewer snacks and had reductions in their BMIs. While most parents don't have access to accelerometers, you can use the same idea — kids only get to watch TV or play video games after they've been active for a set time period.

For older kids, limiting computer use can be tricky since they may complain that they need the computer to do their homework but like Larry, spend most of the time playing games. If this becomes an issue, you can move the computer from the teen's bedroom to a public area and still maintain a two-hour limit on its recreational use.

## Media Literacy 101

Watching television with your child is a great opportunity to correct some of the unrealistic images and falsehoods presented on the tube. For example, when you're watching a commercial glorifying unhealthy foods, you can explain why we rarely eat this food. You can also describe the photographic methods, make-up and clothing tricks that are used to make actresses and rock stars look unrealistically thin.

When you are discussing TV with your child, don't get too critical. Limit yourself to one or two comments per show so that she doesn't feel that you're criticizing her choices. Instead of lecturing her you can have a good time helping your child recognize that much of what she sees on TV is make-believe. When my children were young we would enjoy acting out the commercials, making fun of the exaggerated claims. They can be fun to watch as long as kids recognize that they are no more realistic than Superman flying or Wonder Woman deflecting bullets with her bracelets.

Especially for girls, media images of models and actresses can contribute to body image dissatisfaction that might lead to an eating disorder in adolescence. To reduce this risk, ask your daughter about some of the images she's seen in the program you're watching. "What do you think of (name of actor or actress)?" This will be a chance for your child to verbalize her ideas about the ideal body shape and weight. You can use this to start a discussion explaining how images on TV are frequently unrealistic. Actresses and actors spend hours working on their appearance and have the help of hair stylists, makeup artists, trainers, and dietitians, and if they are still dissatisfied with their appearance they can have the photographer or camera operator modify the image that you see. Discussing the unreality of TV images can help you get started on Step 10.

## Action Plan

1. I will take the TV out of _____'s room. If he complains, I will explain that _____ _____.

2. I will discourage eating while viewing.

3. I will set a limit of _____ hours of TV watching on weekdays and _____ hours on weekends.

4. I will set a limit of _____ hours of playing computer games, X Box, Wii, etc. on weekdays and _____ hours on weekends.

5. I will watch at least part of a program with _____ and have a brief discussion with her about the program (what she thought of the program, liked or disliked, actors and actresses, commercials, etc.)

# Step 10: Help Your Child Have a Positive Body Image, Regardless of His Weight

For kids (and adults), hating your body makes it more difficult to lose weight. Typically when a child doesn't like his body, the motivation to eat healthy and be active DECREASES. He becomes demoralized and may engage in unhealthy eating behaviors. For example, research suggests that binge eating is more likely when a child is dissatisfied with his body. Even if there's no evidence of disordered eating, if your child is unhappy with her body, she'll feel badly about herself when she sees her reflection or steps on the scale. This is distressing and lowers her self-esteem.

When your child looks in the mirror and thinks her "butt" is too big or hates her "flabby" thighs or "poochy" stomach, she is hating part of herself. It's hard to feel good about yourself when there's a part of your body that you find disgusting. Hating your body drains the motivation necessary to make the changes required for weight control. Discouraged, the self-hating, overweight child develops a fatalistic "what's the use" attitude and stops trying.

For parents, it may seem like an impossible dilemma. How can you encourage weight loss without making your child feel badly about his body? It's simple: focus on healthy eating and physical activity rather than on your child's weight. There are many skinny kids that could improve their eating and exercise habits. Everyone, fat, skinny or in the middle, regardless of their weight should develop healthy eating and exercise habits, so you don't need to focus on his weight to encourage positive change.

## How Do You Feel About Your Body?

Although your child will be exposed to negative messages about weight from friends and the media, what parents say and do will have a significant impact on how kids think about their bodies. Research shows that Dad's comments or "good-natured kidding" about weight can undermine his daughter's body image. Likewise, mothers need to be careful about what they say about their own body. When Moms express frustration with their bodies, they are modeling body dissatisfaction to their daughters.

Rosalie, a 46-year-old teacher was about 20 pounds above her ideal weight. She had a lengthy history of yo-yo dieting and was discouraged because even when she lost some weight, she still didn't like the shape of her body. Getting ready to go out with her husband and daughter, Rosalie looked in the mirror, tugged at her dress, and complained, "Nothing helps, my butt is too big." Unfortunately, Brooke, her 11-year-old daughter, was within earshot. When they arrived at the family dinner, her sister complimented Rosalie on her new outfit. Rosalie responded, "Yeah, but I still need to lose 20 pounds." What lesson is Brooke learning from her mother?

Does this sound familiar? Over 90 percent of American women report some dissatisfaction with their bodies and often they teach their daughters to be equally unhappy with their bodies. If you're one of the dissatisfied majority, you need to work on improving your own body image, if for no other reason than to help your daughter. Recognize that hating the way you look does NOT help you lose weight. There are plenty of reasons for losing weight even if you like your body. You would still want to lose weight to reduce your health risks or to be able to do activities that are difficult at a heavier weight.

While you're working on your body dissatisfaction, make sure your daughter doesn't hear you criticize your own body and let her hear you taking some pride in your appearance. If someone compliments you, the best response is, "Thanks," or even "Thanks, I like the way it looks too," instead of, "Yes, but I still need to lose ___ pounds."

Regardless of your child's weight, you need to encourage her to feel good about her body. Surely your child has features that are attractive——nice eyes, a cute smile, or pretty hair. Overweight boys can be handsome, have strong arms, or a nice smile. Help your child feel good about his appearance even if he is significantly overweight. Your child can take pride in her body because it provides pleasure when doing fun things and makes her feel powerful when she uses it to accomplish worthwhile goals.

While encouraging a positive body image, be careful that you don't communicate a mixed message. For example, in several workshops I was giving women described bad feelings after being told, "You have such a pretty face." Think about the implication in that compliment——your face is pretty but the rest of your body isn't. It would have been better to just say, "You're so pretty."

## Spot Reducing

If your child is already unhappy with her body, try to find out which part of her body is causing the most dissatisfaction. For girls, it frequently is the buttocks, thighs, stomach, or breasts. Boys also are concerned that they don't have "six packs" (a flat stomach) or that their muscles aren't big enough. For many kids (and adults), understanding the genetics of weight distribution will help. Simply put,

*You have some control over how much fat will accumulate on your body but you have no control over where it will end up.*

Eating less and exercising more will get rid of some of the fat, but maybe not the fat that you find troubling. This is determined by your genetic makeup ——you've inherited it from your ancestors.

Since childhood I've had a stomach that sticks out, regardless of my weight. When I was heavier, my stomach was bigger, but now that I'm not as heavy, it still sticks out, only not as far. For most of my adult life I've lamented that I don't have a flat stomach. When I first joined a gym, I headed straight to the crunch machine to work on my stomach flab. Using this machine strengthens abdominal muscles. Over several months I gradually increased the amount of weight I was using and eventually was doing 30 crunches with all the weight possible. The result of all this hard work is that I have very strong abdominal muscles behind the fat; my stomach still protrudes. You can't exercise away fat from one part of your body. Likewise, any "spot reducer" gizmo is going to fail.

Sometimes kids (and parents) get discouraged because they're doing everything right but they're still dissatisfied with their thighs, butt, or some other body part. If your child is fixated on a part of her body that refuses to get smaller, she may become discouraged and give up or she may resort to drastic measures like self-induced vomiting. To prevent this, you can help your child understand that she can be attractive and healthy even if she doesn't have a perfect figure. Mrs. L. told Amanda, her 12-year-old daughter:

> All the women in our family have big hips. I have big hips and Grandma and Aunt Sandy also have big hips. Even with my hips, Dad still loves me. You're probably going to have big hips, too, but you're still smart, very pretty, and fun to be around, so boys will like you.

It may also help to explain that just like fashions in clothing change, fashions in body shape change too. For example, looking back in time, 1920's vintage flappers seem silly, not beautiful. Who knows what future generations will think about our current preoccupation with being thin?

## Preparing for Perplexing Puberty

Puberty is a major milestone in your child's life. For boys it's usually a source of pride; he's becoming a man. If your son is one of the first in his group to mature, he'll earn extra status from his friends as his voice deepens and peach fuzz appears on his face. He's likely to be self-confident and may be chosen as a leader of his peer group. Unfortunately, early maturing girls are not so lucky. Frequently girls are embarrassed about their newly rounded shape. Your daughter may try to hide her body from her more angular friends by wearing loose-fitting clothes. Since many girls interpret the physical changes that come with puberty as evidence that they're getting fat, they may intensify their efforts to diet. Since adolescent dieting rarely works, she'll become increasingly frustrated, demoralized and may resort to extreme measures to try to lose weight.

If you've got a young daughter, you can help prevent the body dissatisfaction that often comes with puberty by explaining the anticipated changes well before they arrive. This discussion, along with talks about the inheritance of body shape, can help your child understand that weight and body shape are not just a matter of will power. While being encouraged in their healthy eating and exercise habits, children also need to understand that biology limits how much we can change our bodies. They're more likely to persist with habit change when they have a healthy body image and realistic goals.

## Action Plan

1. Even when I am discouraged about my own weight I will not make negative comments when my children are present.

2. I will occasionally compliment my child's appearance when he is dressed nicely or looks good regardless of his weight.

3. When appropriate, I will explain how heredity determines where fat will accumulate on our bodies and help my child accept genetically determined features.

4. I will discuss the changes that come with puberty before they occur.

5. I will discourage unrealistic weight reduction goals.

# Part III: The Larger Picture

Many parents feel that they're fighting an uphill battle trying to help their children maintain a healthy weight. It's difficult——we live in a fattening environment. If you've been implementing the 10 Steps you've been creating a healthy weight environment at home, but your child still has to deal with the world outside your doors. While you don't have control over what goes on in his school, in your community, or the media and society, you are not completely helpless. In this section I'll describe several approaches to make your child's world less fattening. As a parent you may want to get involved or, at the very least, support these efforts to prevent juvenile obesity.

## Individual Responsibility vs. Public Health

Most people view obesity as merely a matter of will power, or personal responsibility. From this perspective, preventing obesity is straightforward; just eat less and exercise more. But it's not that simple. Eating and exercising are influenced by the child's environment. It's more realistic to look at obesity as a public health issue, rather than as just a matter of individual responsibility, but doing so can be controversial. If childhood obesity is a public health issue, should government get involved in personal decisions about eating and exercise? In addition to education about nutrition, should taxes and regulations be used to discourage junk food consumption? Needless to say, any government intervention will be challenged as depriving us of our freedoms. Food and restaurant groups will decry the intrusion of the "nanny state," and will lobby against government intervention in personal choices.

To understand the benefits and costs of the public health approach, it's helpful to look at the example of cigarette smoking. Before the Surgeon General's Report linking cigarettes with lung cancer, smokers were expected to exert "will power" if they wanted to quit. Once smoking became a public health issue, legislation designed to make smoking more difficult was passed, instead of expecting persuasion to get individuals to quit. Starting with warning labels on cigarette packs, efforts included banning cigarette ads on TV, public health messages describing the hazards of smoking, prohibiting smoking on airplanes, in restaurants and other public areas, and increasing the taxes on cigarettes. These efforts contributed to the marked decline in smoking over the last 20 years, but would a similar approach reduce childhood obesity?

Fighting smoking entailed a long, costly battle with the tobacco industry. Waging a similar battle to prevent childhood obesity will be more difficult. With smoking, the goal is a smoke-free society, but no one is suggesting that we try to eliminate eating to prevent juvenile obesity. Any public health efforts are going to require a more subtle intervention.

Sugar-sweetened beverages are a good place to start since they're one of the most significant contributors to the juvenile obesity epidemic. Sodas, sport and energy drinks have no nutritional value and account for 10-15 percent of the calories consumed by kids and teens.

In 1994, Kelly Brownell, Ph.D., Director of the Yale Center for Eating and Weight Disorders, proposed taxes on snack foods and beverages along with regulations restricting food advertising directed at children. He proposed levying a one-cent per ounce tax on sugar-sweetened beverages. This would reduce consumption by 13 percent and result in a five-pound average weight loss in a year. So far, the soft drink industry has succeeded in defeating soda taxes in Maine, New York and Philadelphia, but as was the case with cigarettes, it's likely that eventually public health concerns will prevail.

## School-based Programs

There are numerous studies demonstrating that school interventions can reduce children's consumption of high fat, high sugar foods while increasing fruit and vegetable consumption. School programs may include mandatory screening of children's BMI, removing vending machines and junk foods from school cafeterias, and educating children about the dangers of being overweight. Although well intentioned, some of these interventions may increase the risk of unhealthy weight control practices and, perhaps, eating disorders. For example, public weighing in school is likely to increase the stigmatization of overweight kids.

Implementing a school program requires great sensitivity. Recall from Step 10 that having a healthy body image helps kids with weight control and reduces the risk of developing an eating disorder. Unfortunately, when teachers, coaches, and school programs focus on weight loss, the message frequently implies that overweight kids should hate their bodies. Instead of an anti-obesity campaign, schools should adopt a pro-healthy body campaign. This approach would minimize stigma and would be helpful for more kids, since many normal weight children would improve their eating and exercise habits. Cutting back on sodas, fast foods and high calorie snacks, while reducing the amount of time spent on video games and watching TV, are worthwhile goals for children regardless of their weight.

As a parent, you can support healthy weight programs while encouraging teachers, principals, and school nurses to eliminate fat jokes, public weigh-ins, and weight loss contests, and promote the inclusion of girls with less than perfect bodies as cheerleaders or in other high profile school positions.

Alice Waters, the founder of Chez Panisse, an elegant restaurant in Berkeley, California, proposed another school-based approach. In 1995 she suggested that a vacant lot at a local middle school be used to plant an organic fruit and vegetable garden. The students plant, tend to the garden, harvest the produce and cook healthy meals in an adjacent kitchen. The program has been so successful that it will be expanded to 15 other public schools. Waters summarized the results of the Edible Schoolyard Program, "...if the kids grow it and cook it, they'll eat it." In nearby Oakland, the non-profit Oakland Food Connection sponsors a similar program for urban high school students. In one year the kids harvested over 150 pounds of produce and brought most of it home to share with their families.

In most schools, there's less opportunity to be active than there was when you were in school. One study found that only a third of high school students attended gym classes at least once per week. This trend is unfortunate since research has demonstrated the benefits of physical activity in school. For example, a Kansas study found that elementary school students who had 75 minutes or more of physical activity showed significantly less increase in BMI after three years. Does your child have the opportunity to be active in gym class or during recess? Even if your child's school has cut back on PE class, there are simple changes to the school environment that can help increase the activity level of students. For example, a study of 15 English elementary schools found that painting school playgrounds with markings that encourage playground games increased physical activity.

<h2 style="text-align:center">What Can I Do?</h2>

While you're using the 10 Steps to create a healthy weight environment at home, consider what's happening at your children's school. One concerned parent in San Jose, California conducted a successful two-year campaign to replace all candy, soda, and junk foods at a middle school with healthier snacks in the cafeteria and vending machines. If you're not that ambitious, you can still have an impact on your child's school. Ask about the lunches served in the school cafeteria. For alternatives to the typical pizza slices and fried chicken nuggets, suggest a salad bar. School personnel can check the "Great American Salad Bar Project" (http://saladbarproject.org) for ideas.

Ask your kids about the opportunity to be active in school. If you find their gym classes or recess activities to be lacking, bring it up at a PTA meeting. Also, you could organize a Walking School Bus (see Step 8). It shouldn't be too difficult to talk to neighborhood parents to get it going. Even if their children aren't overweight, most parents recognize that their children are spending too much time in front of screens and not enough time being active, so they might welcome an activity that gets their kids moving.

Beyond your children's school, there are many ways you can help create a healthy weight environment for all kids. You can work to reduce stigma, discrimination, and bullying that overweight kids experience and help other parents recognize that dieting for kids and teens is counterproductive. You could call or email TV stations to object when they present programs glorifying unrealistically thin body types, mock overweight people, or run commercials for junk foods that are aimed at kids. You can support efforts to create bike paths, outdoor recreation areas or hiking trails in your community. You can back proposals to tax sugary drinks and zoning restrictions to minimize the number of fast food outlets near schools. It's going to take a concerted effort to insure that our kids, and our kids' kids, don't have a shorter lifespan than we do. Implementing the 10 Steps to create a healthy weight environment in your home is a good place to start.

# Recommended Reading

Abramson, E. E. (2006). *Body intelligence: Lose weight, keep it off, and feel great about your body without dieting!* New York: McGraw-Hill.

Bauer, J. (2010). *Slim and scrumptious.* New York: William Morrow.

Wansink, B. (2006). *Mindless eating: Why we eat more than we think.* New York: Bantam.

Waters, A. (2008). *Edible schoolyard: A universal idea.* San Francisco: Chronicle Books.

Zinczenko, D. (2008). *Eat this, not that! for kids!* New York: Rodale.

# Bibliography

Berkowitz, R. I., Moore, R. H., Faith, M. S., Stallings, V. A., Kral, T. V. E., & Stunkard, A. J. (2010). Identification of an obese eating style in 4-year-old children born at high and low risk for obesity. *Obesity, 16 (3),* 505-512.

Birch, L. L. (2002). Acquisition of food preferences and eating patterns in children. In C. G. Fairburn & K. D. Brownell (eds.), *Eating disorders and obesity: a comprehensive handbook (2nd ed.)* (pp. 473-476). New York: Guilford.

Birch, L. L., & Fisher, J. O. (1998). Development of eating behavior among children and adolescents. *Pediatrics, 101* (Suppl.), 539-549.

Birch, L. L., & Fisher, J. O. (2000). Mothers' child-feeding practices influence daughters' eating and weight. *American Journal of Clinical Nutrition, 71,* 1054-1061.

Boynton-Jarrett, R., Thomas, T. N., Peterson, K. E., Wiecha, J., Sobol, A. M., & Gortmaker, S. L. (2003). Impact of television viewing patterns on fruit and vegetable consumption among adolescents. *Pediatrics, 112 (6),* 1321-1326.

Cho, S., Dietrich, M., Brown, C. J. P., Clark, C. A., & Block, G. (2003). The effect of breakfast type on total daily energy intake and body-mass index: Results from The Third National Health and Nutrition Examination Survey (NHANES III). *Journal of the American College of Nutrition, 22,* 296-302.

De La, O. A., Jordan, K., et al. (2009). Do parents accurately perceive their child's weight status? *Journal of Pediatric Health Care, 23,* 216-221.

Dennison, B. A., Erb, T. A., & Jenkins, P. L. (2002). Television viewing and television in bedroom associated with overweight risk among low-income preschool children. *Pediatrics, 109(6),* 1028-1035.

Dietz, W. H. (2002). Medical consequences of obesity in children and adolescents. In C. G. Fairburn & K. D. Brownell (Eds.), *Eating disorders and obesity: A comprehensive Handbook (2nd Ed.)* (pp. 473-476). New York: Guilford.

Diliberti, N., Bordi, P. L., Conklin, M. T., Roe, L. S., & Rolls, B. J. (2004). Increased portion size leads to increased energy intake in a restaurant meal. *Obesity, 12,* 562-568.

Eneli, I. U., Crum, P. A., & Tylka, T. L. (2008). The trust model: A different feeding paradigm for managing childhood obesity. *Obesity, 16(10),* 2197-2204.

Faith, M. S., Leone, M. A., Ayers, T. S., Heo, M., & Pietrobelli, A. (2002). Weight criticism during physical activity, coping skills, and reported physical activity in children. *Pediatrics, 110(2),* 1-8.

Faith, M. S., Scanlon, K. S., Birch, L. L., Francis, L. A., & Sherry, B. (2004). Parent-child feeding strategies and their relationships to child eating and weight status. *Obesity Research, 12(11),* 1711-1722.

Freedman, D. S., Kahn, L. K., Dietz, W. H., Srinivasan, S. R., & Berenson, G. S. (2001). Relationship of childhood obesity to coronary heart disease risk factors in adulthood: The Bogalusa Heart Study. *Pediatrics, 103,* 1175-1182.

Freedman, D. S., Khan, L. K., Serdula, M. K., Ogden C. L., & Dietz, W. H. (2006). Racial and ethnic differences in secular trends for childhood BMI, weight, and height. *Obesity, 14(2),* 301-308.

Goldfield, G. S., Mallory, R., Parker, T., Cunningham, T., Legg, C., Lumb, A., Parker, K., Prud'homme, D.,

Gaboury, I., & Adamo, K. B. (2006). Effects of open-loop feedback on physical activity and television viewing in overweight and obese children: A randomized, controlled trial. *Pediatrics 118(1)*, 157-166.

Gortmaker, S. L., Must, A., Sobol, A. M., Peterson, K., Colditz, G. A., & Dietz, W. H. (1996). Television viewing as a cause of increasing obesity among children in the United States, 1986-1990. *Archives of Pediatric and Adolescent Medicine, 150*, 356-362.

Klesges, R. C., Shelton, M. L., & Klesges, L. M. (1993). Effects of television on metabolic rate: Potential implications for childhood obesity. *Pediatrics, 91*, 281-286.

Levine, J., Baukol, P., & Pavilidis, I. (1999). The energy expended in chewing gum. *New England Journal of Medicine, 341*, 2100.

McConahy, K. L., Smiciklas-Wright, H., Mitchell, D. C., & Picciano, M. F. (2006). Food portions are positively related to energy intake among preschool-aged children. *Journal of the American Dietetic Association, 104(6)*, 975-979.

National Institutes of Health (2010). Serving size card. Retrieved from: http://hp2010.nhlbihin.net/portion/servingcard7.pdf

Newmark-Sztainer, D. (2005). Can we simultaneously work toward the prevention of obesity and eating disorders in children and adolescents? *International Journal of Eating Disorders, 38*, 220-227.

Neumark-Sztainer, D., Story, M., & Fabisch, L. (1988). Perceived stigmatization among overweight African American and Caucasian adolescent girls. *Journal of Adolescent Health, 23*, 264-270.

Ogden, C. L., Flegal, K. M., Carroll, M. D., & Johnson, C. L. (2002). Prevalence and trends in overweight among US children and adolescents, 1999-2000. *Journal of the American Medical Association, 288(14)*, 1728-1732.

Patel, S. R., & Hu, F. B. (2008) Short sleep duration and weight gain: A systematic review. *Obesity, 16(3)*, 643-653.

Richie, L. D., Welk, G., Styne, D., Gerstein, D. E., & Crawford, P. B. (2005). Family environment and pediatric overweight: What is a parent to do? *Journal of the American Dietetic Association, 105(5, Supplement 1)*, S70-S79.

Rideout, V. J., Foehr, U. G., & Roberts, D. F. (2010). *Generation M2: Media in the lives of 8-to 18-year-olds.* Menlo Park, CA.: Henry J. Kaiser Family Foundation.

Staunton, C. E., Hubsmith, D., & Kallins, W. (2003). Promoting safe walking and biking to school: The Marin County success story. *American Journal of Public Health, 93(9)*, 1431-1434.

Stettler N., Signer, T. M., & Suter, P. M. (2004). Electronic games and environmental factors associated with childhood obesity in Switzerland. *Obesity Research, 12(6)*, 896-903.

Stice, E., Cameron, R. P., Killen, J. D., Hayward, C., & Taylor, C. B. (1999). Naturalistic weight-reduction efforts prospectively predict growth in relative weight and onset of obesity among female adolescents. *Journal of Consulting and Clinical Psychology, 67*, 967-974.

Stratton, G., & Mullan, E. (2005). The effect of multicolor playground markings on children's physical activity level during recess. *Preventive Medicine, 41*(5-6), 828-833.

Van Jaarsveld, C. H. M., Fidler, J. A., Steptoe, A., Boniface, D., & Wardle, J. (2009). Perceived stress and weight gain in adolescence: A longitudinal analysis. *Obesity, 17(12),* 2155-2161.

Wright, K. P. (2006). Too little sleep: A risk factor for obesity? *Obesity Management, 2(4),* 140-145.

# About the Author

Edward Abramson, Ph.D. is a licensed clinical psychologist maintaining a private practice in Lafayette, California. He is a Professor Emeritus at California State University, and was the Director of the Eating Disorders Center at Chico Community Hospital. A formerly fat kid and overweight adult, he knows that it's easier to prevent obesity in childhood than it is to lose weight as an adult. He enjoys teaching parents how to help their kids maintain a healthy weight without increasing the risk of an eating disorder. Dr. Abramson is the proud father of two grown active, healthy weight adults but admits that his cat could stand to lose a little weight.

Dr. Abramson is the author of four previous books including *Body Intelligence* and *Emotional Eating* as well as many scientific studies of obesity and eating disorders. Dr. Abramson has appeared on dozens of TV and radio programs including *20/20, Hard Copy,* and *Joan Rivers.* His work is routinely noted in publications including *The New York Times, Good Housekeeping, O, The Oprah Magazine* and *Fitness. Men's Health* magazine called him "the go-to authority on the 'why' of weight gain.

Dr. Abramson has lectured widely throughout the US., Canada, and Europe. He frequently offers continuing education workshops for health professionals and gives keynotes and presentations to parent groups, educators, and the general public.

For more information about workshops and presentations check his website: www.dredabramson.com or email: edabramson.phd@gmail.com.

9 780615 420752